W9-BNL-426

The Wrinkle Cure

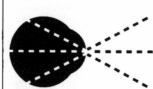

This Large Print Book carries the
Seal of Approval of N.A.V.H.

The Wrinkle Cure

Unlock the Power of **Cosmeceuticals**
for Supple, Youthful Skin

Nicholas Perricone, M.D.

Assistant Clinical Professor of Dermatology
Yale University School of Medicine

Thorndike Press • Waterville, Maine

© 2000 by Nicholas Perricone

This book is intended as a reference volume only, not as a medical manual. The information given here is designed to help you make informed decisions about your health. It is not intended as a substitute for any treatment that may have been prescribed by your doctor. If you suspect that you have a medical problem, we urge you to seek competent medical help.

Published in 2002 by arrangement with Rodale Press, Inc.

Thorndike Press Large Print Senior Lifestyles Series.

The tree indicium is a trademark of Thorndike Press.

The text of this Large Print edition is unabridged. Other aspects of the book may vary from the original edition.

Set in 16 pt. Plantin by Al Chase.

Printed in the United States on permanent paper.

Library of Congress Cataloging-in-Publication Data

Perricone, Nicholas.
  The wrinkle cure : unlock the power of cosmeceuticals for supple, youthful skin / Nicholas Perricone. — [Thorndike large print ed.].
      p. cm.
  Previously published: Emmaus, PA : Rodale, 2000.
  ISBN 0-7862-4236-1 (lg. print : hc : alk. paper)
  1. Skin — Care and hygiene.   2. Skin — Wrinkles — Prevention.   3. Functional foods.   4. Dietary supplements.   5. Antioxidants — Therapeutic use.   I. Title.
  RL87 .P466 2002
      646.7′26—dc21   2002022879

In memory of Dr. Sidney Hurwitz, Clinical Professor of Pediatrics and Dermatology, the Yale University School of Medicine, who served as a guide and role model for my medical career.

Acknowledgments

I would like to thank the many friends and colleagues who have assisted me in my scientific work and/or in the creation of this book, including:

My colleagues at Yale University School of Medicine and my friends and colleagues at the College of Human Medicine, Michigan State University.

My colleagues and friends at the Henry Ford Hospital.

Alan McFarlane for years of dedication and firm belief in my technology.

Dr. Stephen Sinatra for his guidance in the nutritional aspects of anti-aging.

My agent and friend Anne Sellaro for always being there and listening, for finding me the perfect publisher, and for her never-ending wellspring of creative ideas.

Nada Lantz, of Lantz-a-Lot, whose expertise continues to make all the difference in the world, and Bob Krasnow for his wisdom and solid support. Also, to Tonya Giver of Lantz-a-Lot.

My editor, Nancy Hancock, for her unmatched skill in translating twenty years of scientific research into an entertaining as well as instructive book that everyone can understand.

Maria Verel, whose kindness and generosity of spirit are matched only by her great skill as a makeup artist/designer.

Matt Van Leeuwen for his confidence, flair, and outstanding talent.

Sherree Crute, who so beautifully integrated my words into a cohesive, easy-to-read book.

Julie Logan for reviewing this manuscript.

Kevin Hogan, a good friend and positive supporter.

My scientific colleagues and sources of inspiration and knowledge, including Imre Zs.-Nagy, whose work has been the focus of my research; Lester Packer, one of the world's finest scientists, whose research has been absolutely essential to my own work; Dr. Denham Harmon, for the original thinking that made all of this happen; and Linus Pauling, who guided my vitamin C research with unequalled wisdom and insight.

Dr. Jeffrey and Dr. Harry Hurley for their friendship and support.

Olga Marko for her valuable scientific protocols.

Debbie Barela and Dale Crighton, Mary Krinsky.

Steve Goldstein, for years of friendship.

Richard Rubenstein, for seeing the vision and bringing it to the world.

Joe Grace, Mary Thornton, Chim Potini, Nancy Fogg Johnson, Laurie Bush, Chris Molinari, Zoe Gilman, Dana Darty, Jan Marini, Stevie Wilson, Steve Bock, Shashi Batra, and Hillary Weidert.

Nordstrom, the first retailer who believed in NVPerricone, and to Sephora and Saks Fifth Avenue, our newest retail partners.

Joan who prepared this manuscript as well as my other dedicated staff members, Gee, Amy, and Linda.

Lynn Russell for positive words of support.

To the incomparable professionals at Rodale, Neil Wertheimer, vice president and publisher; Cindy Ratzlaff, director of publicity; and to the entire Rodale sales and marketing, production, and design staffs, and to Hugh O'Neill for getting this project off the ground.

My mother and father for their love and guidance.

To Nicholas, Jeffrey, and Caitlin for their love and patience.

And a special thanks to my beautiful Madeleine for urging me to write this book.

Contents

Chapter 1

Beautiful Skin

for Life

Wrinkled, sagging skin is *not* the inevitable result of growing older. It's a disease, and you can fight it. You can look your best, feel your best, and enjoy beautiful skin and optimum health every day of your life, provided you start right now. And you don't need expensive, invasive plastic surgery to do it.

After nearly two decades of scientific research, I have discovered a revolutionary, all-natural approach to preventing the signs of aging by putting nature's most powerful nutrients to work for your skin.

In my dermatology practice in Connecticut, I use cosmeceuticals to treat a whole host of skin problems, from acne, uneven pigment, dark circles, and poor skin tone to fine lines, sagging skin, and loss of radiance — problems that often come with age. My hundreds of patients come from all walks of life, from teenagers to grandfathers, from soccer moms to celebrities, and I'm proud to say that they consistently leave my office

15

with great results. You can, too. By following my program, you can have smooth, radiant, youthful skin well into your forties, fifties, sixties, and beyond.

Of course, beautiful skin on the outside begins with good health on the inside. Think about it: have you ever seen an unhealthy person with a flawless complexion and a radiant glow? Of course not. Beautiful skin doesn't come in a bottle. Although your skin may appreciate the care and attention you lavish on it from the outside — creams, gels, and gentle soaps — it will suffer dearly from the damage you cause on the inside if you don't get enough sleep, smoke, drink too much alcohol, don't eat properly, and don't take essential vitamins, including A, C, and E.

Good Nutrition for a Great Complexion

My daughter Catie is only two, but she's already on her way to a lifetime of good health and beautiful skin. Every morning for breakfast, she climbs into my lap, asks for her special toddler-sized "Catie fork," and digs right into my breakfast, a morning meal of grilled salmon, fresh blueberries and strawberries. No sweetened cereals or toaster pastries for Catie. In fact, she likes my breakfast so much that some days I leave for work hungry.

Our unusual breakfasts are just one part of the health and nutrition plan I've developed during 15 years of research into what keeps our skin and bodies young and vital. My interest in nutrients and healthy foods may seem unusual in a dermatologist, especially at a time when surgery, laser, and other high-tech treatments are the focal point of much of the work done in my profession.

I like to think I've always been a little ahead of the curve. In today's world of health food superstores and daily fitness workouts, it may seem hard to believe that doctors were once resistant to accepting nutrition as a critical part of preventive medicine. But back in 1979, when I entered medical school at the Michigan State University College of Human Medicine, the study of nutrition (and the beneficial effects of exercise, for that matter) was virtually unheard of.

My own fascination with nutrition was sparked during my undergraduate days, before I entered medical school. I had always suffered from sallow, acne-plagued skin, allergies, and fatigue, so I started reading everything I could find on the sub-

Cosmeceutical Countdown: Four Weeks to a Fabulous Face

Jeannie W., 45, seemed nervous and upset when she first came to me for a consultation. Not long ago, she told me, she'd been making a purchase in a local department store when the clerk asked for her senior citizen discount card. Annoyed, Jeannie pressed the clerk for a reason. She was told, matter-of-factly, that it was company policy to ask for a senior's card whenever there was any question about a customer's age.

Jeannie was devastated. To make matters worse, her college reunion was coming up in four weeks. She'd been looking forward to attending, but now she didn't have the confidence to go.

I examined Jeannie's face. It showed a moderate amount of sun damage, especially around the eyes and forehead. She had deep folds above her mouth, some loss of tone around her jawline, some sagging in her upper eyelids, and dark circles under her eyes. Her light complexion appeared sallow and dull. Overall, she looked older than she actually was.

What she needed was an intense program that would produce dramatic results in just a short time. First, I put Jeannie on a diet rich in vegetables, fruits, lean meats, and salmon. Next, I started her on a complete topical regimen including:

- High-potency alpha lipoic face cream, designed to increase circulation. It would tighten her pores, even out her complexion, and give her a healthy glow in only three to four days.

- Alpha lipoic eye therapy along with vitamin C ester eye therapy. Both compounds act as anti-inflammatories to bring down some of the puffiness and help erase the dark circles under the eyes. Lipoic acid eye therapy contains *DMAE,* short for *dimethylaminoethanol,* a nutrient that improves skin tone and lifts sagging eyelids. DMAE works very rapidly: Jeannie could actually see changes within 20 minutes. The improvement was even more marked after three weeks, and the result was a more youthful, wide-eyed look.

- Concentrated vitamin C ester cream containing DMAE. Used on her face and neck at night, this nutrient combination helped to reduce sagging, to tighten the skin around her jawline and to smooth the skin in her neck.

After two weeks of treatment, Jeannie returned to my office showing remarkable changes in her face — and her attitude. Her complexion glowed, and the dark circles under her eyes had diminished by half. Her sagging eyelids were tighter, and her eyes were wider. Her jawline was firmer, her pores were tighter, and her complexion in general was softer and more plump. She was amazed and delighted with the changes in her looks.

Jeannie was doing beautifully, but we still had two weeks to go — and more to do — before her reunion. She told me that she planned to wear a gown that revealed her back and shoulders. I prescribed a body toning lotion containing DMAE, instructing her to apply it to her shoulders, back, and legs. It made her skin appear smooth and porcelain-like, and it also helped to reduce dimpling in the thighs. I also recommended an "instant face-lift" in the form of a product that contains high concentrations of DMAE and tightens and tones the skin. It lasts for about 24 hours after it's applied.

Finally, I recommended a special eating regimen beginning 72 hours before the big event, including a 6-ounce serving of fresh grilled salmon, a salad of romaine lettuce dressed with lemon juice and olive oil, and daily servings of fresh cantaloupe. These foods would help erase fine lines and make her skin moist and smooth. With that,

Jeannie was ready for her reunion.

I got a call from her two weeks after the event. She was ecstatic. She'd received dozens of compliments from classmates who told her how young she looked. And she was sure it would be quite some time before anyone asked for her senior citizen card!

---

ject — which, at the time, pretty much meant everything written by Linus Pauling, Ph.D., a strong proponent of vitamin C, and nutritionist Adele Davis. I began experimenting with vitamins on my own, and the results were gratifying. My skin and allergies improved, and I had much more energy.

After graduation and a short stint in the army, I became director of the Connecticut branch of the Muscular Dystrophy Association. I continued to keep a careful eye on nutrition research, and I was particularly intrigued by anecdotal evidence that muscular dystrophy patients seemed to improve by taking high doses of vitamin E. I began looking into vitamins as therapeutic agents for chronic, incurable diseases.

When I entered medical school, however, my interest in nutrition made me an eccentric. My classmates thought I was nuts because I popped vitamins after meals and bundled up to go running in the dark, cold mornings of Michigan winters. In those days, medicine meant intervention, not prevention, and our professors brooked no equivocation. I'll never forget the afternoon I arrived for a lecture to find my classmates passing around a sheaf of papers and trading furtive whispers in one corner of the classroom. At first I thought they had a contraband copy of an exam. It turned out to be a research paper on homocysteine, vitamin B, and heart disease prevention — research that would be widely accepted in the medical community 15 years later and go on to help save lives. But at the time, we students understood that such a thing had to be hidden from our professors. Any show of interest meant that we weren't serious medical students.

Fortunately, I wasn't deterred by medical school, and my own experiences only fueled my interest. As a firm believer in the powers of vitamin C, I kept my energy high during my grueling class schedules by taking powdered doses mixed with juice throughout the day. One day, after a particularly long run, I came home with a badly sunburned face. On a whim, I mixed a bit of the vitamin C powder with water and put it on my face. It soothed the irritation immediately. Although it hardly qualified as a scientific experiment, this was my very first evidence that vitamin C could help stop inflammation.

The Cosmeceutical Alternative

When I entered my first residency, at Yale University, I began to investigate the role of nutrients in health and disease seriously. I continued my research at the Henry Ford Medical Center in Detroit. By then, doctors and scientists in many areas of medicine had recognized the importance of nutrients in both healing and maintaining good health.

I have been conducting scientific research into the use of nutrient cosmeceuticals in skin care for nearly 15 years. My firm belief in nutrients is at the foundation of my work. I am very concerned about the disappointing results of some of the invasive treatments that are widely used to correct the problems associated with aging skin. Before coming to me, many of my patients have chosen to undergo surgical procedures, such as face-lifts and dermabrasions, to correct skin problems. They were unprepared for the inherent limitations of such surgical techniques, and they were disappointed by the outcomes. For people with dark or even pale brown skin, for example, scarring and uneven pigment problems are common after surgery or laser treatments. Face-lifts can produce a tight, artificial effect, no matter how skilled the surgeon. And I confess I'm often astounded by the amount of money my patients have spent on products that offer little more than gorgeous packaging and expert marketing.

During the course of my research, I uncovered a wider range of skin care options. I've developed a groundbreaking approach based on nutrient *antioxidants,* a concept we'll explore later in this book. Antioxidants can impede and even repair the damage to skin cells that comes with aging. Soft, radiant, younger-looking skin is the gratifying result.

The term *cosmeceutical* refers to a skin treatment that provides added benefit beyond a simple cosmetic or moisturizer. Cosmeceuticals are not considered a medication and therefore are not regulated by the FDA.

My cosmeceutical program includes these components:

- Vitamin C esters
- Alpha lipoic acid

- DMAE, an acronym for the nutrient *dimethylaminoethanol*
- Tocotrienols, a high-potency form of vitamin E
- Alpha hydroxy and beta hydroxy acids

These components are gentle, all-natural, noninvasive — and best of all, they work. By combining my cosmeceutical program with healthy living habits, you can achieve beautiful skin for the rest of your life.

Chapter 2

Understanding Aging Skin

Just as softness is the signature of a rose at first bloom and smoothness is the hallmark of a swath of finely spun silk, supple, glowing skin is one of the most memorable characteristics of a child's face. No matter how many fine lines and furrows you accumulate by your fourth or fifth decade, you entered this world with a virtually flawless complexion.

So just what is responsible for transforming that baby-smooth skin into the crepe and crinkles of middle age? Some of the answers lie in the nature of skin itself. Our skin works incredibly hard for us, but we tend not to work hard for it. In fact, we tend to take it for granted.

We shouldn't. The skin is an organ, just like our hearts or our livers. Like any vital organ, it performs a long list of life-sustaining tasks. It regulates body temperature. It's the body's sensor, registering pressure, temperature, and pain. It's a barrier against the elements and a shield against bacteria, viruses and other external threats to our health. It's also the body's mirror: When we're chronically fatigued, poorly nourished, or physically or emotionally stressed, our skin reacts. Premature aging is one consequence of failing to give our skin the care and attention it needs.

The Skin You're In

Our skin is our body's first line of defense. As such, it's easily damaged, both by external causes — sunlight, air pollution — and internal factors, such as cigarette smoke or a diet that lacks nutrients, particularly antioxidant nutrients such as vitamins C and E.

To truly understand what our skin is up against — and to grasp its intricacy — consider its structure. Your skin consists of three basic layers: the epidermis, the dermis, and a fat layer.

The epidermis. This is your skin's outer layer. The very outer surface of the epidermis, called the *stratum corneum,* is a protective coating of dead skin cells that forms when fresh cells made in the skin's deeper layers push their way to the surface, flatten, and die. This layer is thinner than a sheet of tissue paper.

The stratum corneum is sloughed off continually as new cells take its place. But as we age, this sloughing process slows down. In a young person, cell turnover occurs about every 28 to 30 days. By the time we're in our sixties, the process takes 45 to 50 days, which is one of the reasons our skin loses the freshness of youth as the years go by. Although the stratum corneum is essentially "dead," it serves an extremely important function: It helps your skin hold in moisture and oil.

Basal cells, which produce new skin cells, are at the bottom of the epidermis. The epidermis also contains cells called *melanocytes*. These cells produce melanin, which determines the color of your skin. Although we all have about the same number of melanocytes, the actual tone of your skin depends on your skin's unique amount and concentration of melanin, a trait you inherit from your mom and dad.

The dermis. You might call the dermis, which lies under the epidermis and makes up 90 percent of the thickness of your skin, the skin's nerve center — it's where much of the skin's important work is done. The dermis contains nerve receptors, which are sensitive to pressure (soft kisses, the stroke of a feather), temperature, and pain; sweat glands, sebaceous glands (which produce skin-protective oil), hair follicles, and blood vessels.

The sweat and sebaceous glands in the dermis help produce your skin's acid mantel, a thin coating of oil and perspiration that helps protect you from infections, bacterial and fungal. This acid mantel is an effective barrier. Unfortunately, we often unwittingly strip it away through the use of harsh soaps, which disrupt your skin's natural balance of acidity and alkalinity (called pH).

The dermis also contains a dense meshwork of collagen and elastin, two types of protein that give your skin its strength and elasticity. More about these in a moment.

The fat layer. Under the epidermis and dermis is tissue composed mostly of fat. The fat layer serves to insulate and protect your inner organs and acts as a sort of cushion that helps keep the skin plump and smooth.

Why Our Skin Ages

One of the questions my patients ask most often is: "Does the skin on the face age faster than the skin on the rest of the body?" My answer: It appears to. The truth is, it's the way we treat our skin — not the aging process — that "ages" facial skin the most.

Scientists explain it this way: There are two types of aging, *intrinsic* and *extrinsic*. Intrinsic (internal) aging is the rate of aging that occurs with the passage of time. Extrinsic (external) aging is intrinsic aging compounded by external causes such as sunlight, air pollution, and inflammation caused by harsh detergents, rough treatment, cosmetics, and disease processes.

To understand the difference between intrinsic and extrinsic aging, you need only look at the skin on your face versus, say, the skin on your hips or your upper thighs. The prime culprit of extrinsic aging? Sun exposure. Most 50-year-olds, for example, can easily see the difference in skin that's been exposed to sunlight for years (such as the skin on their faces, necks, arms, chests, and lower legs) and skin that's been protected by clothing (such as the skin on their buttocks and torsos). The exposed skin is generally more wrinkled and discolored and less taut than the unexposed skin.

Compounding extrinsic damage is the fact that with age your body's ability to repair itself slows considerably. When we're 11, our cells can repair themselves nearly perfectly from damage, but at age 50, the aging process begins to accelerate because we no longer have that ability for perfect repair. The question is: Why?

The Free-Radical Theory of Aging

Theories as to how and why we age abound. The pioneering work of researcher Leonard Hayflick, Ph.D., paved the way for the idea that aging is no mysterious event that occurs at random. Rather, it is a pre-programmed process that begins at the cellular level. And through his work it eventually became clear that finding ways to reduce or eliminate cell damage could significantly affect the aging process.

But among all the theories of aging, it's the free-radical theory — proposed by Denham Harman, M.D., Ph.D., at the University of Nebraska back in the mid-1950s — that is perhaps the most universally accepted. Chapter 4 covers Dr. Harman's work in detail, but the theory is so essential to understanding how and why we age that it deserves mention here.

In a nutshell: Free radicals are oxygen molecules that have lost an electron in interactions with other molecules. As a result, these molecules are extremely unstable, or reactive. In their quest to "heal" themselves, free radicals steal electrons from other, healthy molecules, creating more free radicals in the process, damaging cell components.

Although free radicals are entirely natural — they're a by-product of normal bodily processes, like breathing air or digesting food — they're also extremely treacherous. Because every time free radicals seek to stabilize themselves, they damage healthy cells. Worse, free radicals aren't just manufactured by our own bodies. They're also unleashed by external factors, including sunlight, cigarette smoke, and air pollution.

What does all this have to do with aging skin? A lot.

Collagen, a protein, is one of the substances that gives our skin its youthful suppleness and tautness, and it is especially susceptible to damage from free radicals. Because collagen stays in our skin for years, free radicals attack it mercilessly. This sustained attack leads to a chemical change called *cross-linking* — a fancy way of saying that free radicals wreak havoc on the protein molecules that make up our skin (actually, our whole bodies).

Normally, collagen molecules "slide" over one another, which gives skin its softness and resiliency. But once they've been damaged by cross-linking, they become stiff and inflexible, and that condition tends to make the skin look "old."

Although there are many causes of free-radical damage to the skin, one of the most insidious is sunlight. What happens when the sun hits your skin is enough to make you shudder.

First, as you stroll in the park on a bright, sunny day, the molecules in your skin absorb sunlight. Presto — free radicals are activated. The sunlight also activates an enzyme that breaks down fats in skin cells. This fat breakdown produces a chemical called *arachidonic acid,* the precursor to molecules that can inflame the skin. And we now know that these inflammatory molecules accelerate the aging of skin.

Meanwhile, inside your skin cells, free radicals activate molecules called *transcription factors*. These are chemical "messengers" that signal cellular DNA to produce proteins that tell your cells what to do.

Transcription factors are harmless little molecules that float around inside of our cells unless they are activated. If we go into the sun and sunlight strikes our skin, free radicals are created. These free radicals turn on the little innocent molecules called transcription factors, causing them to migrate to the center of the cell called the nucleus. Once they get to the nucleus, they turn on DNA for production of various chemicals; in the case of transcription factor NFk-B these chemicals are pro-inflammatory which, of course, is harmful to the cell, and accelerates the aging process. When stimulated by ultraviolet light, these transcription factors can turn on AP-1. AP-1 begins producing collagen-digesting enzymes that can leave tiny defects in the skin. Gary Fisher, Ph.D., a research dermatologist at the University of Michigan, termed this process "microscarring," and it is the birth of a wrinkle.

In other words, a wrinkle is created by these tiny little scars that are formed when sunlight-activated AP-1 turns on this collagen-digesting enzyme. Sunlight is not the only way that AP-1 can be turned on, however. Powerful antioxidants like alpha lipoic acid can also activate AP-1, with the reverse effect. When AP-1 is turned on by alpha lipoic acid, the collagen-digesting enzyme attacks only the damaged collagen, and can actually help repair the tiny scars, thus improving or erasing a wrinkle.

Antioxidants to the Rescue

Happily, our skin has allies in its continuing fight against free-radical damage. Through my work, I've discovered that certain nutrients called *antioxidants* (a group that includes certain vitamins, amino acids, and other natural substances) can stop or even reverse free-radical damage and put an end to subclinical inflammation and micro- and macroscarring — or at least repair a good deal of the damage these processes can cause over the years. You'll learn more about the power of antioxidants in the next few chapters.

As you read, you will come to see that *The Wrinkle Cure* offers more than a plan for maintaining youthful, glowing skin. It also offers a complete anti-aging diet and supplement program that will help you combat the aging process throughout your body.

How can I make such promises? Years of research. After dedicating much of my career to understanding the connection between aging, free-radical damage, inflammation, and the healing effects of oral and topical antioxidant therapy, I realized two very exciting things: First, we do not have to age like our parents. We can hold on to our vitality and looks well into our later years. Second, plastic surgery isn't the only way to keep the aging process at bay. With the proper care, you can have fabulous skin in your forties, fifties, sixties, and beyond.

These promises are not based on my assumptions or observations alone. In the following chapters, you will be given your own opportunity to read about the research and understand how you can use certain nutrients, including antioxidants and amino acids, to heal, protect, and nurture your skin so that it continues to look, feel, and act young and healthy.

The Beauty Clock

Ever stand inches away from the mirror, closely examining your face because you're sure you see a wrinkle that was absolutely not there the day before? Relax. Time does not march on quite that fast.

In fact, time is not your skin's greatest enemy. The natural aging process gets a tremendous push from

- Sun exposure
- Cigarette smoke (inhaled or secondhand)
- Environmental toxins
- A nutrition-poor diet, especially one lacking in vitamins A, C, E, and folic acid yet high in fat and salt
- Excess alcohol consumption
- Stress
- Harsh soaps or detergent-based moisturizers
- Sleep deprivation

But even if you manage never to leave the house without sunscreen or to inhale a puff of smoke, your skin will follow this process:

Dryness. The skin's oil glands reduce their production significantly after about age 30, and the loss continues over the years.

Sun damage/loss of skin tone. Melanocytes begin to burn out when you reach your late thirties and forties, reducing the skin's ability to fight sun damage and often causing uneven pigmentation.

Thinning. At about age 40, the dermis and the skin's fat layer begin to thin. The process picks up steam after your 50th birthday. The unhappy result: sagging and the loss of the plump, youthful softness. The loss of the fat layer also makes the skin more fragile and likely to abrade.

Loss of firmness. In the dermis, cells called *fibroblasts* constantly replenish our skin's supply of collagen and elastin. Fibroblasts lose their ability to function over the years, resulting in the reduction of collagen and elastin.

Diminished immune response. The skin is home to Langerhan's cells, receptors for the immune system that register the presence of foreign agents and toxins. Without them, you are less likely to get a quick warning signal when you come in contact with irritants.

Reduced ability to repair damage. Overall, the body loses its ability to repair free-radical damage, so changes in the cells become more pronounced, accelerating aging.

Loss of temperature control. Sweat glands also slowly lose their ability to function, which makes it harder for your body to regulate itself and register heat and cold.

Chapter 3

Taking Care
of Your Skin

None of us can completely escape the physical effects of living long and interesting lives, but each of us will field the slings and arrows time sends our way very differently — and that's especially true when it comes to our skin.

As you have just learned, we all have the same, basic skin structure, but each of us has a different genetic code. The rules and regulations permanently imprinted on your DNA determine whether you'll get crow's-feet or brow furrows, have a tendency for acne, and how easily you'll tan or burn. If you have alabaster skin with invisible pores, for example, my guess is you sailed through high school with only a blemish or two, but you may have more difficulty fending off sun damage. If, on the other hand, you have brown skin in any range of tones from café au lait to ebony, you may have struggled with excess oil and breakouts for years, but because your skin is more resistant to sun damage, you may be well into your fifties before you see your first fine line.

The bottom line — each skin tone and type has its rewards and challenges, and that is why choosing the right skin care for your skin type is crucial if you want to get the best results. To give your skin this care, you need to identify two basic attributes about your skin: its tone and its type.

Skin tone is, well, the color of your skin — alabaster white, golden olive, ebony black, or any shade in between. Skin tone is determined by the content of melanin, the pigment that gives skin its color. The more melanin your skin contains, the darker it is.

Melanin also determines how well the skin can withstand sun damage and irritation. The fairer your skin, the less melanin it contains — and the more vulnerable it is to sun damage (and sun-related discoloration and wrinkles). Olive and yellow skin contain more melanin, making them more impervious to sun damage and premature skin aging. Dark brown or ebony skin contains the most protective melanin of all. (But make no mistake: Dark skin can and does burn.)

When we talk about *skin type*, we mean whether your skin tends to be dry, oily, or a combination of both. Why do we need to know our skin type? Because skin products aren't one-size-fits-all. Cleansers or astringents formulated for oily skin are likely to parch and irritate dry or sensitive skin, and oil-based cleansers, moisturizers, or makeup can cause bumps and breakouts on oily skin.

Regardless of your skin's tone or type, the bottom line is this: A little care goes a long way. For most people, a skin care program that emphasizes natural products can maximize the good qualities of their complexions by improving color, clarity, and smoothness, while minimizing or resolving problems such as discoloration or fine lines.

Treat Your Skin Tone Right

Most of the differences that exist among the various shades of skin can be attributed to melanin content. In addition to establishing the skin's color, it also controls a person's ability to resist sun damage and recover from irritation or inflammation. Dermatologists judge the skin's light sensitivity by using a color scale that ranges from one to six. People who are at one on the scale are fair-skinned people who always burn and cannot tan. People at six have dark brown skin that can resist sun damage longer than other types of skin. A Latino or Middle Eastern person would fall at about four or five on the scale.

Following are descriptions of the unique characteristics of each skin tone.

White Skin

People with the lightest complexions (Caucasians of all shades, but especially people of Irish or Nordic descent) are far more susceptible to skin damage and photo-aging from repeated exposure to sunlight. Melanin literally absorbs the sun's rays, so people with little or no melanin in their skin have few natural defenses.

The Upside: White skin scars and discolors less easily than other skin tones. So it generally responds well to cosmetic procedures such as dermabrasion, deep acid peels, and cosmetic surgery of all sorts, including face-lifts.

The Downside: Because it's thinner and contains less melanin than darker skin, white skin is more vulnerable to sun damage, ruddiness (redness), and broken blood vessels and capillaries, especially along the cheeks and the sides of the nose. White skin is also prone to rosacea, a form of severe skin inflammation that can mimic acne's pimples and is often characterized by broken blood vessels. Finally, white skin is more susceptible to precancerous and cancerous skin lesions. The fairer the skin, the more vulnerable it is.

Case Study: At 51, Ellen, a fair-skinned, blue-eyed blonde, came into my office with problems typical of fair white skin: brown splotches caused by sun damage and fine lines and wrinkles. Her jawline had also started to sag. She was convinced that her only option was cosmetic surgery. Not so.

Although a face-lift can dramatically improve the skin's *firmness,* it can't improve the skin's *texture.* So all a face-lift would do is pull Ellen's lines and wrinkles into a new position.

By contrast, antioxidant therapy can help improve the actual health of the skin as well as slow the development of new lines and furrows. I put Ellen on aggressive antioxidant therapy, which included high-potency products such as alpha lipoic acid (ALA) and vitamin C ester. Topical vitamin C ester, an antioxidant, can help increase the skin's production of collagen, thereby helping to thicken the skin.

Within three months, Ellen's brown splotches and fine lines had begun to fade, and her skin appeared firmer, thanks to the vitamin C ester therapy. She happily decided to put off laser therapy and a face-lift for a while.

The Bottom Line: Although antioxidant therapy can help repair the punishing rays of the sun, it can't completely eliminate the skin-damaging effects of a lifetime of unprotected sun exposure. So I'll caution all readers: Use at least an SPF-15 sunscreen. Every day. Before you apply your morning makeup. Or at least wear a foundation that contains SPF-15 sunscreen. Coat your neck, chest, and hands with sunscreen, too. The thinner, more delicate skin on these areas is ground zero for sun damage.

Brown Skin

There are vast differences between brown and white skin in terms of how each tone of skin responds to damage from the environment, other irritants, and how it heals.

The Upside: Brown skin contains more melanin than white skin. So it's less likely to sustain sun damage — and more likely to remain smooth and wrinkle-free longer. Brown skin also tends to be oilier; it contains a greater density of sebaceous (oil) glands. This extra oil helps keep lines and wrinkles at bay. As a bonus, there's some evidence that brown skin is more elastic and tends to stay firmer longer.

The Downside: Brown skin is extremely susceptible to inflammation. In fact, in brown skin, a mild case of acne can trigger an extreme inflammatory reaction. That's because in skin with a high melanin content, inflammation triggers the production of chemicals that swiftly attack and break down the elastin in skin. This process can lead to visible scarring, changes in pigment, and, sometimes, large, raised scars called *keloids*. This inflammatory response is also why black skin may be left with a dark spot — called *post-inflammatory hyperpigmentation* — from a minor scratch or abrasion, or even one pimple. (Black skin can also *lose* pigmentation — a condition called *hypopigmentation*, or *vitiligo* — but this condition is less common.)

Many men with brown skin find themselves plagued by ingrown hairs and razor bumps, especially after shaving. It is estimated that approximately 60 percent of black men have a condition called *pseudofolliculitis barbae* — a very fancy term used to explain the inflammation process that occurs when curly hairs work their way back into the skin and produce shaving bumps. Just about any man with skin that has a significant melanin content is at risk for razor bumps.

Case Study: Judy, a 39-year-old African-American patient of mine, came to my office suffering with some tough skin problems — facial scarring caused by acne and discoloration from eczema.

Her condition had become even more severe after she applied benzoyl peroxide, the popular acne medicine. It left brown marks in areas where she hoped it would clear her complexion. Judy didn't realize that slathering irritants such as harsh soaps or strong acne medicines on brown skin could actually increase inflammation and hyperpigmentation. She was learning the hard way that in order to keep brown skin looking its best, you have to be very selective about the products you choose.

Many of today's state-of-the-art treatments — lasers, deep peels, dermabrasion, and, of course, all forms of plastic surgery — involve causing some initial injury or inflammation to the skin. In pigmented skin, this injury can result in scarring, instead of an enhanced appearance. Even products such as Retin-A (a derivative of vitamin A that causes inflammation) or strong acid solutions may cause damage to extremely sensitive individuals. When used in moderate doses, however, alpha hydroxy acids (which are also antioxidants, by the way) can balance uneven pigment in brown skin or solve other problems. (See "Helpful? Harmful? Overrated?" on page 64.)

Judy had active acne breakouts on some parts of her face and multiple dark acne scars on her cheeks, forehead, and chin. The eczema had spared her face, but it had left patches of dark brown to gray pigment on her lower legs. Given her reaction to benzoyl peroxide, it was clear that she was very sensitive to irritants and allergens. Like many people with brown skin, she needed a treatment that was exfoliating, yet healing and gentle. The dermabrasion or deep acid peeling that some doctors might use to remove acne scars in white skin would have produced disastrous results on Judy's delicate complexion.

I treated her with a combination of cortisone creams (to stop further discoloration from her eczema), and gave her a mild alpha hydroxy acid lotion to apply twice daily to her discolored legs. I also treated her face with topical antibiotics (to stop her breakouts) and followed with alpha lipoic acid to treat her acne scars. Within three months her face had cleared dramatically, and she was also looking younger (a pleasant side effect of the topical antioxidants). The pigment on her lower legs had begun to even out and return to her natural, healthy brown tone.

The Bottom Line: Despite its abundance of protective melanin, brown skin needs tender, loving care. Avoid skin products that work primarily by irritating or inflaming skin, such as astringents. Use acne medications with caution, and avoid those that contain more than 2.5 percent benzoyl peroxide. (Absolutely avoid the 5 or 10 percent concentrations.) Also, be aware that although Retin-A (an acidic form of vitamin A) and Renova (which contains the Retin-A molecule but in a very mild base) work beautifully to fade lines and wrinkles on white skin, they can discolor brown skin if not used in the right strength. But brown skin can tolerate treatment with alpha hydroxy acids (AHAs), a group of natural acids derived from fruit, milk, and other natural substances that work as gentle exfoliants. When used conservatively, alpha hydroxy acids can correct uneven pigment in brown skin. (For more information, see chapter 8.) Throughout this book, you will see how antioxidant therapy can help brown skin recover from discoloration, overactive oil glands, and other problems.

Light Brown or Yellow Skin

Even small amounts of melanin can have a tremendous impact on how your skin behaves. This is most evident in people from Asia and the Mediterranean. The complexions of people of Asian descent range from light beige to deep yellow, while people of Italian, Middle Eastern, or Mediterranean descent have a distinctive darker white skin with a golden undertone. This "extra" melanin gives Mediterranean and Asian skin many of the good qualities — and problems — of brown skin.

The Upside: Asian skin is more resistant to sun damage, for example, than white skin, but, unlike brown skin, the pores tend to be tiny, giving the skin a very smooth appearance. Mediterranean skin, by contrast, tends to be thicker and oilier. This may mean bigger pores, but less susceptibility to sun damage and the prospect of fewer wrinkles down the road.

The Downside: Both Mediterranean and Asian skin can appear sallow, or yellowish. Carefully adhering to a healthy diet that hydrates the skin is the best prescription for many medium-skinned patients. Drinking a minimum of eight to ten glasses of water per day and eating plenty of antioxidant-rich fruits and vegetables are important components of staying healthy for everyone, but for people of Asian and Mediterranean descent these guidelines are especially helpful for avoiding problems with sallow skin tone. Mediterranean skin can also be oily with occasional blemishes. In addition, any type of inflammation (from chemicals, mild trauma, or other irritants) can quickly lead to discoloration. On close examination, the extreme inflammatory response common to Asian skin is similar to that of brown skin.

Case Study: Lia, a 54-year-old Asian-American patient who came to me a few years ago, was upset about the fine wrinkling, dull skin tone, and puffiness that she had developed in middle age. She was sure that only surgery and facial liposuction could help her.

After examining her carefully, I explained that alpha lipoic acid, vitamin C ester, and other treatments would greatly improve her appearance. She was so skeptical that she said she would buy me dinner at the restaurant of my choice if my cosmeceutical program really worked.

I said, "You've got a deal," and I quickly got her started on a regimen of alpha lipoic acid cream containing DMAE with 15 percent vitamin C ester to begin reducing the fine lines and puffiness (another consequence of inflammation) around her eyes, and alpha lipoic acid to apply to her entire face. I asked her to call me the minute she saw any results.

I was delighted when my office phone rang the very next morning. It was Lia informing me that the anti-inflammatory effects of the eye therapy were already working, and she just could not believe that she was already seeing less puffiness under her eyes. Within three to five days she reported a healthier glow to her skin, which basically meant that the alpha lipoic acid had helped increase her circulation, reducing some of the sallowness of her complexion. You see, in addition to reducing inflammation, alpha lipoic acid has a unique effect on an enzyme in the skin called *nitric oxide synthase,* which controls circulation: the alpha lipoic acid increases the amount of this enzyme and just lights up the skin. Within three months, her fine lines began to diminish, and Lia declared that she was happy with the results. She still owes me dinner, but her willingness to stick with a natural, antioxidant program rather than opt for surgery was enough of a reward for me.

Her decision may also have spared her some disappointment. Remember, Asian skin is similar to brown skin in how it responds to inflammation and abrasion. After undergoing the surgical procedures Lia had in mind, her skin tone might have worsened because the healing process could have created uneven pigmentation.

The Bottom Line: Both Mediterranean and Asian skin can appear sallow, or yellowish. Carefully adhering to a healthy diet that hydrates the skin is the best prescription for many medium-skinned patients. Drinking a minimum of eight to ten glasses of water per day and eating plenty of antioxidant-rich fruits and vegetables are important parts of staying healthy for everyone, but for people of Asian and Mediterranean descent these guidelines are helpful in avoiding problems with a sallow skin tone.

Treat Your Skin Type Right

Dry Skin

Although that tight, parched feeling in the skin can be age-related, *dry* skin can also be caused by using a cleanser that's too harsh or a moisturizer that's not rich enough for your skin's needs. A gentle skin care routine can help make even the driest skin more supple and radiant.

Cleansing: Dry skin needs a gentle cleanser. Fortunately, there are plenty to try: There are "superfatted" soaps — often called beauty bars — that contain emollients such as olive oil or lanolin, and there are milky liquid cleansers and tissue-off cleansing creams.

Moisturizing: The drier your skin, the more hydrating ingredients your moisturizer should contain. Pick a product formulated with glycerin, hyaluronic acid, or dimethicone. These ingredients slow down moisture loss during the day, preventing further dehydration. Or go the natural route and just slather your face with olive oil. (Of course, avoid this treatment if you're prone to acne.) Use olive oil as a before-bed treatment. But be aware that although it makes a great salad dressing, olive oil can't protect your skin from the sun.

Cosmetics: Look for oil-based foundations, blushers, and powders. Oil-based makeups will have words such as *hydrating, nourishing,* and *moisturizing* in their names. Choose cream or cream-powder blushers, because they will make your skin look dewy; powder blushers will emphasize lines and wrinkles.

Sun Protection: Dry skin produces less oil than other skin types, so it's more vulnerable to inflammation. Use an SPF-15 sunscreen — or a moisturizer with added sunscreen and antioxidants — year-round.

Dry Skin: The Rules

Do . . .
- Use a mild, soap-free liquid cleanser or "superfatted" cleansing bar to wash your face at night. In the morning, just splash your face with warm water.
- Select moisturizers formulated with glycerin, hyaluronic acid, or dimethicone, which delay moisture loss, preventing further dryness.
- Apply moisturizer when your face and body are still damp so that you "lock in" the moisture.
- Use oil-based foundations and cream or cream-powder blushers — the oil they contain will help soften fine lines and wrinkles.

Don't . . .
- Wash your face with harsh soap. Ever.
- Use grainy cleansing products or buffing pads.
- Forget to apply an SPF-15 sunscreen to your face, neck, and chest every day.

And don't be stingy: Use a marble-sized amount of sunscreen to cover your face and two "marbles" to cover your neck and chest.

Oily Skin

If you have oily skin, consider yourself blessed. The oil you bemoan now is a built-in lubricant that will benefit your skin as you grow older.

Of course, you may have to deal with a shiny nose and greasy cheeks now. The solution: Don't fight it, control it.

Cleansing: If you're using harsh, detergent-based soaps and alcohol-laden astringents to dry up the oil, stop. Immediately. Over time, these products can damage your skin — and they may encourage already overactive oil glands to step up production. Try an oil-binding liquid or gel cleanser formulated for oily skin. And avoid "superfatted" soaps that contain oily ingredients such as cocoa butter, cleansing cream, or lanolin. The most effective oil control cream to date is a new release called Clinac O.C., which is a molecule that absorbs oil and breaks it down to harmless substances. This technology comes from a chemical originally designed to scoop up oil spills in the ocean. When added to a cream, Clinac O.C. can reduce facial oil, minimizing facial shine. This product works for many hours and can be used with makeup. It does not exacerbate acne and is nonirritating.

Moisturizing: Depending on how oily your skin is, you may not need a moisturizer

Oily Skin: The Rules

Do . . .

- Cleanse your face twice a day — in the morning and before bed — with a mild liquid cleanser formulated for oily skin.
- Use astringents no more than once a day. Better yet, don't use them at all. Use Clinac O.C. (available at drugstores) to soak up excess oil.
- Choose an oil-free or oil-in-water moisturizer if you feel you need to use a moisturizer.
- Use oil-free or oil-blotting foundation and powder and powder blusher to stop oily shine and head off breakouts.
- Use an oil-free sunscreen with an SPF of at least 15 every day.

Don't . . .

- Overscrub your skin. Oil is your skin's protective barrier.
- Cleanse your face more than twice a day — but you may cleanse once more if you work out.
- Develop an astringent addiction.
- Use moisturizer if you don't need it.
- Keep slapping on powder to mop up oil — your skin will look chalky.

at all. Or you may only *think* you need one, because you've been using harsh cleansing products that have stripped the oil from your skin. But if you think you need one, go for moisturizers that contain *humectants* (ingredients that attract and hold water), such as glycerin and sodium pyrrolidone-carboxylic acid (PCA). These ingredients trap water in your skin without producing a greasy shine. Also choose a lotion. They're lighter than creams and tend to contain less oil, so they won't clog pores.

Cosmetics: Opt for oil-free and water-based foundations. They won't add extra oil to an already oily complexion. Other options are oil-blotting foundations and powders, which delay shine by soaking up excess oil. Use powder rather than cream blushers.

Sun Protection: Many people with oily skin shy away from sunscreens, fearing that the oil they contain will trigger breakouts. Now there's no excuse: Oil-free sunscreens were made for you. They can keep your skin safe from solar assault without adding extra shine.

Combination Skin

Caring for combination skin is a balancing act: You need to moisturize the drier areas, typically the cheeks, while treating the oiliness of the oilier areas such as the forehead, nose, and chin (the so-called *T-zone*). But that doesn't mean you have to have a tackle box of skin care products. Just a few basic products will do the trick.

Cleansing: There are plenty of cleansers for combination skin on the market. Look on the label for the phrase "for normal/combination skin." If your T-zone is very oily, you can use an astringent — but only once a day. Use it more, and you're setting yourself up for dry, flaky skin.

Moisturizing: The last thing you want to do is make your already oily T-zone even oilier. So use a moisturizer only where you need it — on combination skin, that's usually the cheeks. If your under-eye area is dry, use a cream specifically formulated for this delicate skin. Eye creams contain preservatives that keep them sterile and prevent eye infections.

Cosmetics: Try a water-based foundation first. But if your T-zone is extremely oily, consider opting for an oil-free foundation. Apply it after you use a moisturizer on drier areas.

Sun Protection: Opt for an oil-free SPF-15 sunscreen, or an oil-free moisturizer with added SPF-15 sunscreen.

The Gender Gap

When it comes to differences in skin, this is one case in which the differences between the sexes can truly be chalked up to nothing more than biology. The variations in male and female skin begin deep down in the very structure of the skin's fat layer and dermis. Women have thinner skin than men because testosterone — the dominant male hor-

---

Combination Skin: The Rules

Do . . .
- Choose cleansers formulated for combination skin; they're gentle on dry areas, such as the cheeks, and tougher on oily cheeks, nose, and chin.
- Apply moisturizer only where you need it, but slathering it on your T-zone may lead to breakouts.
- Use water-based or oil-free foundation.

Don't . . .
- Use a different cleanser or moisturizer for different parts of your face — it's a waste of time and money.
- Forget to use a sunscreen with an SPF of at least 15 every day. Use a product formulated without oil, if you like.

---

mone — causes male skin to be thicker. In addition, women's oil glands secrete slightly less than men's; therefore, women are more likely to experience dry skin.

As we grow older and our hormone levels begin to change, the differences in male and female skin become even more dramatic. In late middle age, men lose testosterone and women lose estrogen, resulting in thinner, more fragile skin for people of both sexes. In women, however, the drop in hormone activity is more dramatic, and it has a greater effect.

When women enter menopause, they experience a drop in estrogen levels, causing their skin to become more thin and dry. The oil glands begin to slow their production of natural emollients that keep the skin soft. This is the time of life when the skin becomes a less efficient barrier against irritants, allergens, and bacteria. Thinner skin is more susceptible to a type of inflammation called *dermatitis* and more vulnerable to trauma and infections.

The problems associated with menopause can be addressed with hormone replacement therapy, an option women may want to discuss with their gynecologist. Estrogen affects the skin because there are receptors for estrogen in the skin's cells. The estrogen sends messages to the skin's cells that probably contribute to maintaining healthy collagen and other factors. Oral or topical estrogen (creams) can help female skin avoid the changes that come with estrogen loss.

All of these changes mean that for women, keeping the skin moist and hydrated is extremely important. The best way to do this is to follow some very old-fashioned advice: Apply moisturizer directly after bathing, while your skin is still damp, to lock in water.

Thanks to its thickness, male skin tends to be low maintenance — but as a result men tend to take their skin for granted. As a matter of fact, as just about any wife can attest, men are much less likely to go to the dermatologist, wear sunscreen, or even bother using moisturizer. This means that dozens of guys will forfeit their natural protection against wrinkles and dry skin simply by neglecting themselves. In my practice, I have consistently performed more surgery on a type of skin cancer called basal-cell carcinoma on the faces, ears, and necks of men, than on women.

Throughout this book you'll find lots of anti-aging strategies. A sneak preview begins with alpha hydroxy acids (a type of

Getting Skin-Specific

This chart is a very basic guide to the types of problems that are most common in certain skin types. Use this information to

Skin Type	Risks
White	Sun damage
Brown	Inflammation, severe scarring from surgery, uneven pigmentation after abrasions or lasers
Beige or yellow	Moderate inflammation, sometimes sallow; fine lines; uneven pigmentation from abrasive procedures
Female	Premature thinning, dryness, and sun damage
Male	Neglect, leading to possible higher rate of skin cancer and skin damage

Getting Skin-Specific

better understand how the antioxidant treatments discussed in the next few chapters can

Rewards	Best Anti-Aging Treatments
Small pores, fewer breakouts	High-dose alpha lipoic acids, vitamin C, alpha hydroxy acids
Resists sun damage, resists wrinkling and sagging	Mild alpha hydroxy acids and alpha lipoic acids
Smallest pores, resists sun damage	Alpha lipoic acids, hydration, vitamin C, antioxidant-rich diet
Gets better care	Alpha lipoic acids, vitamin C, alpha hydroxy acids, hormone therapy, moisturizer, sunscreen
Thick, resists sun damage and dryness	Alpha lipoic acids, vitamin C, moisturizer, sunscreen

Helpful? Harmful? Overrated?	
Product or Ingredient	**Helpful**
Alpha Hydroxy Acid	At proper percentages (usually 5–10%), if it doesn't cause irritation. On brown skin, small areas should be tested to determine levels that can be tolerated
Cleansers	If they remove oil and makeup without drying
Collagen-Based Creams	Not applicable
Copper Peptide Complex Skin Cream	For aging skin and as anti-inflammatory, if proper percentage of active ingredient is present
Elastin Products	Not applicable

Harmful . . .	Overrated . . .
Not applicable	Not applicable
If they contain harsh alkalis	Not applicable
Not applicable	Because the collagen molecule cannot penetrate skin and is useless
Not applicable	Not applicable
Not applicable	Because the elastin molecule cannot penetrate skin

Helpful? Harmful? Overrated? — Continued	
Product or Ingredient	**Helpful . . .**
Eye Creams and Gels	If they contain nonirritant anti-inflammatories or antioxidants
Eye Makeup Removers	Not applicable
Facial Masks	If used to achieve hydration
Hypoallergenic Products	Not applicable
Moisturizers, Basic, with Petrolatum or Mineral Oil	For normal to dry skin
Moisturizers, with Coenzyme Q_{10}	Because they have anti-oxidant/anti-inflammatory effects

Harmful . . .	Overrated . . .
If they contain petro-latum or oils that can migrate onto the eye	If they are standard moisturizers that claim to remove dark circles
Because some products sting the eyes	Because your normal cleanser can clean off eye makeup, but some products are good makeup removers that aren't irritating
If they cause irrita-tion or are used more often than once a week	For facial rejuvena-tion
Not applicable	Because even though they probably contain no fragrance and fewer allergens, there is no guarantee that these products will not cause allergic reactions
If used on oily skin	Not applicable
Not applicable	Not applicable

Product or Ingredient	Helpful . . .
Helpful? Harmful? Overrated? — Continued	
Moisturizers, Oil-Free	For oily and/or acne-prone skin
Moisturizers, with Oil/Noncomedogenic	Because proper use does not cause acne
Renova (same active ingredient as Retin-A but in a more emollient and less irritating base)	If used on a regular basis
Retin-A (prescription based)	For reversal of photoaging (sun damage) and for patients with acne
Retinol/Vitamin A–Based Cosmetics	If used long-term
Sunscreens	If SPF (sun protection factor) is 15 or higher
Toners	Not applicable

Harmful?	Overrated?
Not applicable	For normal/dry skin (moisturizers with oil are better)
If overused because it can clog pores	Not applicable
If used in conjunction with sun exposure	Not applicable
If it is overirri- tating or if it is used with subsequent sun exposure	Not applicable
If the compound is present at too high a level because it may cause irritation	If the compound is present at a low level and/or not properly stabilized
If used instead of avoiding sun exposure	If used as protection from long sun exposure
If they overdry; not recommended for dry skin types	For pore cleansing

Helpful? Harmful? Overrated? — Continued	
Product or Ingredient	**Helpful . . .**
Vitamin C/ L-Ascorbic Acid	Not applicable
Vitamin C Ester/Ascorbyl Palmitate	Because they act as anti-inflammatory and are stable

Harmful . . .	Overrated . . .
If it causes irritation, which increases inflammation	If active ingredient is present at a low level, or if no active ingredient is present due to instability
Not applicable	Not applicable

antioxidant), which can normalize the uppermost layer of the skin — the stratum corneum — allowing it to hold on to moisture longer. Topical vitamin C ester, which is also an antioxidant, can help pump up thinning skin by increasing its production of collagen. Alpha hydroxy acid can also thicken the skin if it's used regularly. Therefore, a mixture of vitamin C ester and alpha hydroxy acid would make a great anti-aging formula for female skin. But it's still no substitute for the right diet. I cannot overemphasize the importance of drinking eight to ten glasses of water a day and eating a diet rich in antioxidants and vitamins for keeping fragile female skin looking its best.

Chapter 4

How Skin Cells Age

Free Radicals and the Inflammation-Aging Connection

Cruise any department store cosmetics counter, and you'll probably be astounded by the claims on all those sparkling bottles, jars, and vials. The language of beauty has always been filled with fantastic promises and grand declarations. From the earliest days when "vanishing" creams (basically, just moisturizers) guaranteed flawless, eternally youthful skin, until today when virtually every product ensures that it will erase the signs of aging, consumers have been told that there are thousands of ways to hold on to firm skin, smooth out fine lines, and look youthful forever.

Unfortunately, precious few of these claims are true. The harsh reality is that many products offer only limited, short-term benefits.

That's not to say that over-the-counter

skin treatments can't do your skin some good. Many companies produce high-quality emollient and exfoliant formulas that can temporarily smooth the skin's surface or increase its ability to maintain moisture. But again, these are superficial, short-term gains. The only long-lasting solutions to the problems of aging skin are those products and treatments that have been scientifically tested and proven to penetrate to where the aging process actually takes place: in the deeper layers of the skin.

Today there are only a handful of such treatments. The antioxidant and nutrient-based program that I have created provides the most advanced treatment available. Throughout this book you will be introduced to the latest research and the patients who have benefited from putting this research into action.

At the core of my work — and that of several other scientists — are antioxidants, or, more specifically, topical antioxidant preparations formulated to exact specifications so that they can penetrate deeply into the skin. To understand how these preparations work, you must first understand the source of the problem that they attack. In this chapter, we'll look at that source — free radicals — and at the theories that made it possible for me and others in the field of dermatology to bring about the antioxidant revolution in skin care.

Understanding Free Radicals

When it comes to aging, it's not Father Time that's public enemy number 1. It's the very busy, very nasty little molecule called the free radical.

Our cells use oxygen to produce energy. In the process, they generate *free radicals* — unstable oxygen molecules created during such basic metabolic functions as circulation and digestion. Free radicals are also produced by sunlight, by toxins such as pesticides, and by cigarette smoke and air pollution. In your body, free radicals literally bounce about, attaching themselves to other atoms and molecules, whether they're wanted or not. Ridding yourself of them is impossible, because they're an unavoidable by-product of daily living.

Free radicals may sound aggressive, but they are actually just searching for a little company. You see, all molecules want to have a pair of electrons in their outer orbit. Most of the free radicals encountered in our bodies come from oxygen. Therefore, these are called reactive oxygen species because they lack an electron in the outer pair of the molecular orbit, and are looking for a second electron to complete their pair. Therefore, any molecule, such as oxygen, that is lacking an electron in the outer orbit is unstable because it wants to join up with anything close to it.

Unfortunately, much like an out-of-control guy in a singles bar, free radicals get into lots of unhealthy relationships and do their unsuspecting partners — other molecules and atoms — a good deal of harm.

Free radicals can damage virtually every part of a cell, including the nucleus, where DNA, the body's unique genetic blueprint, is produced. They can also harm the fats inside cells. In fact, many scientists believe that free-radical damage is one of the primary causes of aging and age-related diseases such as heart disease, cancer, Alzheimer's disease, and arthritis. If they take the extra electron they need from the collagen molecules in our skin, the result is that the collagen becomes damaged. When the collagen becomes damaged, the skin gets discolored and stiff and loses elasticity. The end result is that free radicals sap our skin of its youthful appearance.

The Theory That Started a Revolution

The first scientist to truly understand how much damage free radicals wreak on our cells was Denham Harman, M.D., Ph.D., who first proposed the free-radical theory of aging way back in 1956. According to Dr. Harman's theory, aging is a result of the damage free radicals do to all the molecules of the cell, including fats, proteins, and DNA. This theory led scientists to believe that most of the damage caused by free radicals centered in the DNA within the cell's nucleus, which then caused a faulty translation of DNA, resulting in accelerated aging.

With all this cell damage going on, the next question that needed to be answered was: How do our cells survive at all? Researchers discovered that one of the reasons that most of us enjoy long, healthy lives is that the body has developed its own unique defense system for fighting free radicals. As you may have guessed by now, this defense system is powered by antioxidants. Antioxidants prevent free-radical damage simply by giving these wildly out-of-control molecules the electron partners they seek. Once the antioxidant joins with the free radical, the free radical no longer attempts to latch on to the various components of other cells. So antioxidants really work by making the free radical harmless.

You may have come to know antioxidants as vitamins. That's because some of the most powerful ones are vitamins such as E, C, and beta-carotene. Others, however, occur naturally inside the human body. These include enzymes (substances that help two or more chemicals interact) with complex names such as glutathione, catalase, and superoxidedismutase that can stop free radicals in their tracks.

The next, and most obvious question is: If antioxidants are in the body and they stop free radicals, why do we age at all? The answer is that it's all a matter of balance. Our bodies have the ability to make antioxidants, and we can replenish them to some degree with supplements and vitamin-rich foods. But under certain conditions, such as prolonged exposure to sunlight or ingestion of toxins such as cigarette smoke, so many free radicals can be produced that the body's antioxidant system is overwhelmed and the free radicals once again move about unchecked. Scientists refer to this process as *oxidative stress,* and it may be occurring in your body at this very moment.

Research has proved that supplementing

the body's supply of antioxidants can keep oxidative stress to a minimum, or at least slow it down considerably. These findings are behind nutritionists' suggestions that we load up on antioxidants each day. Doctors are still debating the merits of this approach, but so far it does not seem to be the complete answer to putting an end to aging and disease processes.

Protecting Cells
from Free-Radical Damage

Although Dr. Harman's work was a critical first step, and subsequent research was adding to our knowledge, significant pieces of information were still missing from the free-radical puzzle. As I set out on my quest to come up with a solution to the problems of aging skin, I quickly concluded that I needed to know much more about exactly *how* free radicals damage cells.

I next turned to the research of Imre Nagy, M.D., a Hungarian scientist who has dedicated much of his career to understanding the aging process.

Like Dr. Harman, Dr. Nagy agreed that free radicals were the root cause of general aging and age-related diseases. But he offered a twist on Dr. Harman's theory: that although free-radical damage was the ultimate cause of aging, most of the damage was to the *outer* layers of the cell, called the cell plasma membrane. It sounds like a subtle alteration of the free-radical theory, but its implications were immense.

Until Dr. Nagy's theory emerged in 1978, scientists believed that free radicals did most of their damage to the *interior* of the cell, and that it was damage to cellular DNA that caused cells to age. Because DNA is the key to our genetic "blueprint," they reasoned, free-radical damage to DNA resulted in the cell's inability to repair itself and, therefore, the physical declines observed as we age.

But Dr. Nagy analyzed DNA from cells taken from people as old as 100. When he isolated these cells and checked their ability to reproduce, the DNA replicated perfectly. In other words, the DNA was *not* damaged — even in people as old as 100. So DNA damage couldn't be the root cause of aging.

Imagine that a cell is like a soccer ball full of jelly. The rubber portion of the ball would be the cell plasma membrane; the jelly inside is the inner portion of the cell. Dr. Nagy's breakthrough — called *the membrane hypothesis of aging* — was realizing that free radicals did most of their damage to the outer layer of the cell — in our analogy, the rubber exterior of the ball. His hypothesis was that free radicals are drawn to areas that have the greatest density of molecules, since those areas are the richest potential source of electrons, and since the cell membrane has the greatest concentration of molecules, it would be the primary target of the free radicals. Again, think of the soccer ball filled with jelly; the outside is densely packed; the inside is more fluid.

Once the cell membrane becomes damaged by free radicals, according to Dr. Nagy's theory, it becomes unable to let nutrients in and wastes out. In this scenario, wastes and salts, such as potassium, begin to take up increasing amounts of space within the cell. As a result the cell's water supply is pushed out, and the cell becomes dehydrated.

Perhaps the biggest implication of this finding concerns our notion of how exactly to protect cells from free-radical damage. Since the outer portion of the cell is mostly fat, we need a fat-soluble antioxidant to go to that area to protect it from free-radical damage. However, scientists erroneously believed that most of the important damage was being done in the interior of the cell —

which is water-soluble. Therefore, they opted for the use of water-soluble antioxidants — but this type of antioxidant was not capable of protecting the most vulnerable portion of the cell.

Once Dr. Nagy had made the link between cell dehydration and free radicals, he began to investigate the possibility that certain antioxidants could somehow prevent cellular dehydration. He proved that adding antioxidants specifically designed to penetrate cell membranes could repair cells and increase their ability to retain water.

Dr. Nagy probably did not realize it at the time, but his discovery made it possible for doctors like me — and others in the field of dermatology — to bring about the antioxidant revolution in skin care. In many ways, both of these visionaries — Drs. Harman and Nagy — are responsible for the direction my research has taken over the past 12 years. They gave me the basics. The tools I needed to genuinely understand how I could create treatments that could prevent and reverse the signs of aging in skin. Throughout the next few chapters, you will see these great scientists' theories at work in a comprehensive nutrition and skin care program that is the first of its kind in the world.

Free Radicals and Inflammation

Free radicals are without question the central players in the aging process. But there is another natural phenomenon that affects aging — inflammation.

When you think of inflammation, you may envision skin redness, swelling, or irritation. But the type of inflammation that contributes to much of aging — called *subclinical inflammation* — is actually invisible to the naked eye. When I attempt to explain this to my patients, I always get a look of surprise. Most people probably have never been told that inflammation regularly exists throughout the body in various forms and to various extremes.

Inflammation — both subclinical and visible — can be triggered by a wide variety of external factors such as the ingestion of toxins (cigarette smoke, for example), the presence of an infection, or excess exposure to ultraviolet radiation, which results in sunburn.

What is the relationship between free radicals and inflammation? When free radicals damage a cell, they cause inflammation. Antioxidants scoop up free radicals, preventing the breakdown of fats in the cell plasma membrane, and preventing the production of arachidonic acid and pro-inflammatory chemicals. In addition, antioxidants such as alpha lipoic acid can prevent the activation of transcription factors that direct the cell nucleus into producing pro-inflammatory chemicals. It is interesting to note that all antioxidants — including vitamins C and E — act as anti-inflammatories. However, not all anti-inflammatories are antioxidants. An example is ibuprofen, a nonsteroidal anti-inflammatory agent that has no antioxidant capability.

Some of this free-radical damage takes place in the cell membrane layer called the lipid (fat) bilayer that makes up the cell plasma membrane. The fats (lipids) from this bilayer can be broken down by a special enzyme called phospholipase A2, which is activated when the skin is traumatized or exposed to sun or chemicals. This enzyme then produces arachidonic acid, which in turn is oxidized into chemicals that produce inflammation. That inflammation, in turn, produces more free radicals. It becomes clear, then, that inflammation and aging are intimately connected.

Another cause of inflammation at the cellular level was identified through anti-aging research. It has been established that when these inflammatory chemicals move into the interior of the cell, certain proteins — among them the "transcription factor" NF Kappa B — are switched on, leading to further inflammation inside the cell. This inflammation accelerates the destruction of the cell — and the aging process. My inflammation theory, coupled with Dr. Nagy's membrane hypothesis, represent important breakthroughs in our understanding of the roles and functions of the cell plasma membrane in the aging process.

The Final Frontier

As vital as the theories of Dr. Harman and Dr. Nagy were to my own work, I knew that I had to make one more discovery before I could create antioxidant preparations specifically to treat aging skin.

I needed to figure out how to get the antioxidants out of the test tube and deep into the skin.

As you'll see in the coming chapters, I have devised topical solutions that allow antioxidants to penetrate the skin. Because these solutions are more than just cosmetics, but not quite pharmaceuticals, the term *cosmeceutical* was created to convey their uniqueness.

Now that you understand the full story of the research behind *The Wrinkle Cure*, let's see the miracle of antioxidants at work. I'm going to begin with the treatment that grew out of my earliest discovery — how to make use of a very special form of vitamin C that fights facial lines.

Chapter 5

Vitamin C

Ester

An All-Star Antioxidant

What do a pineapple, a persimmon, and a luscious, ripe strawberry have in common? They're all jam-packed with an ingredient that can take years off your looks — vitamin C. That's right. The stuff that we take for granted because it's packed into every carton of orange juice and a staple in health food stores was, until a very short time ago, one of the unknown substances when it came to banishing wrinkles and fine lines. Thanks to research I conducted just a few years ago, however, it's now been established that vitamin C — in the proper form — can restore a smooth surface and a youthful glow to aging skin.

The Antioxidant Avenger

As you have seen in preceding chapters, vitamin C is an antioxidant — a substance that vanquishes free radicals, those vicious little molecules that irreparably damage our cells and accelerate the aging process. Vitamin C is one of the trio of all-star antioxidants; the other two are vitamin E and alpha lipoic acid.

What makes vitamin C so wonderful? At the root of vitamin C's restorative powers are its antioxidant properties. Here's just an overview of the role this crucial nutrient plays in our health.

It gooses the immune system. Vitamin C strengthens the body's white blood cells, our chief defense against invasion by bacteria and viruses. Nobel Prize–winning scientist Linus Pauling, Ph.D., believed that supplemental vitamin C could work wonders on immune function. And, indeed, research suggests that people who don't get enough vitamin C are far more vulnerable to a variety of infections and illnesses from colds to cancer.

It helps give us energy. Vitamin C also aids in the production of other essential body chemicals. One of these, called L-carnitine, is essential in producing energy. L-carnitine transports fats into the mitochondria, where the fats are converted to energy. A vitamin C deficiency can cause cells' levels of L-carnitine levels to drop, making it harder for cells to oxidize fats to create energy.

It's essential to the nervous system. Vitamin C also helps produce neurotransmitters, the brain chemicals that help the nerves in the central nervous system (which guide the brain) and the nerves in the peripheral nervous system (which direct muscle movement) communicate. Without this ability to communicate, we can't think clearly or move our bodies.

That's a pretty impressive résumé — and I haven't even mentioned the mountains of studies that suggest that vitamin C also protects against heart disease, cataract formation, and other diseases associated with aging.

As you'll see in the following section, vitamin C's amazing powers of restoration extend to the skin, too — including aging skin.

How Vitamin C Saves Your Skin

Vitamin C is essential for the production of collagen, the strong connective tissue that, essentially, holds us together. Without collagen, we'd literally "fall apart," because this protein holds our skeletons together, attaches our muscles to our bones, and keeps our organs and skin in place.

But vitamin C also works near miracles when it comes to healing inflammation. Here's just one example.

During my pediatric training at Yale Medical Center in New Haven, Connecticut, a group of physicians was researching the effects of vitamin C on asthma, a condition caused by a form of lung inflammation. These researchers found that when vitamin C was administered in large doses to folks with asthma — adults and children alike — these people experienced a reduction in their incidence of acute attacks.

The scientists made two other important discoveries: first, that vitamin C hinders the production of a chemical called *arachidonic acid,* which causes inflammation; second, that vitamin C actually converts the arachidonic acid from a pro-inflammatory chemical into a group of less harmful substances.

This research had important implications for my own work. Lung tissue isn't the only part of the body that can be damaged by arachidonic acid. This chemical also plays a role in the formation of psoriasis and the microscarring that leads to the formation of — you got it — wrinkles.

From Failure to Hope

I had to see if applying vitamin C to the skin could help alleviate some of the skin's unique forms of inflammation — specifically, psoriasis and sunburn. So I asked some of my patients who suffered from these conditions to apply a solution of water and vitamin C to the affected areas. The topical C did seem to help ease redness and pain — but not as much as I'd hoped. Back to the drawing board. One day I had a major epiphany. The problem was not the vitamin C itself, I thought. It was the vitamin's *solubility*.

The solubility of a vitamin — that is, whether it dissolves in water or in fat — determines which part of a cell that vitamin can enter. With antioxidant vitamins, solubility also determines which part of a cell the vitamin can protect from free radicals.

The natural form of vitamin C, L-ascorbic acid, is water-soluble. That means that it can gain admission only to the *inside* of a cell, which is mostly water. So although L-ascorbic acid concentrates in the interior of the cell, it cannot prevent free-radical damage on the outside of a cell. What's more, L-ascorbic acid is very acidic, which makes it quite irritating to the skin. It also

A Scurvy Lot

In this land of plenty, getting enough dietary vitamin C isn't difficult — if we eat lots of vitamin C–rich fruits and vegetables, such as strawberries, tomatoes, and red bell peppers.

But centuries before research found that vitamin C is vital for disease prevention, British sailors all over the world often fell prey to scurvy, a horrendous disease that caused slow wound healing, bleeding gums and tooth loss, pneumonia, and eventually death.

While at sea, sailors ate virtually nothing but preserved meats. (It's hard to get fresh fruits and vegetables when you're stuck on a ship.) A long ocean voyage could — and often did — wipe out half the entire crew.

The amazing thing about scurvy, though, is that you can reverse the condition almost instantly by having several servings of vitamin C-rich foods. Sailors were eventually saved from scurvy when someone thought to add fresh limes to their diet (hence their nickname "limey") during those long months at sea.

breaks down rapidly, losing its potency within 24 hours.

So I began a new search — for a form of vitamin C that could be applied to the skin and would be more effective in preventing free-radical change. My research led me to a substance called ascorbyl palmitate, also known as *vitamin C ester*.

The Breakthrough: Vitamin C Ester

Vitamin C ester is composed of L-ascorbic acid — basic vitamin C — joined with a fatty acid derived from palm oil, called palmitic acid. The chemical bond between an acid and an alcohol is called an *ester bond*. The addition of a small amount of palm oil to the vitamin C molecule may not seem very important, but it was the key to making vitamin C an ideal skin treatment. The first, important change I saw when comparing vitamin C ester to L-ascorbic acid was that the ester was not acidic. The compound is totally nonirritating and can even be placed on an open cut without causing stinging. This is important, because when I applied the L-ascorbic acid form of vitamin C to sunburn, the irritant (pro-inflammatory) effects of the acid tended to counteract the anti-inflammatory activity of the nutrient.

L-ascorbic acid also had one other, very significant drawback: it caused something called a *fenton reaction*. When vitamin C in the form of L-ascorbic acid comes in contact with iron (and your skin is loaded with iron), it produces a dangerous type of free radical, the hydroxyl, that, I began to believe, was responsible for the redness and irritation L-ascorbic acid stimulates when it's left on the skin. In short, vitamin C in the form of L-ascorbic acid did more harm than good when it came to repairing damaged skin.

Another important quality of vitamin C ester is that unlike its acidic cousin it is fat-soluble, which means that it can easily be absorbed into the skin. Also, as a fat-soluble substance, vitamin C ester can penetrate the thin membrane that encases a cell — the cell plasma membrane — which is also primarily fat. In effect, vitamin C ester offers maximum protection against free radicals at the exact spot that they wreak the most damage — the outer portion of the cell.

The increased absorption of vitamin C ester has actually been measured by scientists at Proctor & Gamble. They were able to show that vitamin C ester is absorbed much more quickly and achieves levels ten times higher in the skin than L-ascorbic acid.

Another great advantage of vitamin C ester is its stability. Unlike L-ascorbic acid, it can be mixed into creams and lotions and keep its potency for months — even years — without turning rancid.

Was this, finally, the perfect "skin vitamin"? I thought so. But to make sure, I conducted more studies.

To test my theory, I tried healing sunburns again. Using an artificial ultraviolet light source, I produced small sunburns on the forearms of men and women. I then had them apply one of two creams. One cream contained vitamin C ester; the other did not. The subjects reapplied the creams every four hours.

Within a day or two, the burns treated with the vitamin C ester were almost completely healed. The burns treated with the "dummy" cream stayed red for several days longer. These findings strongly suggested that vitamin C ester was successfully battling the free radicals that create the pro-inflammatory arachidonic acid.

I conducted a second study — this time, to see whether vitamin C ester would have any effect on psoriasis. Patients suffering from psoriasis received either the vitamin C ester cream or a placebo cream. After eight weeks, it was apparent that the psoriasis was somewhat improved in those subjects who had received the vitamin C ester, as opposed to those who had used the lotion alone (the placebo).

I was fortunate to have help from the research of the brilliant cell biologist Olga Marko, Ph.D., who found that vitamin C ester helps stimulate the growth of fibroblasts, the cells that help produce collagen and elastin in human skin. This finding gave me a clue that vitamin C ester could boost collagen production and provide a more youthful appearance.

Youth in a Jar

By this time I was convinced that I was on my way to developing one of the first antioxidant-based anti-aging skin treatments. I was so sure of my findings that, that same year, 1987, I began to patent the process that makes it possible to use vitamin C ester in skin treatments.

But what was most gratifying was witnessing the incredible results that vitamin C ester produced in my patients.

Take Patricia, for example. These days she's a New Jersey–based mom of three boys. But she had grown up in southern California, the original land of the sun worshipper — and her skin had paid the price.

"I'm a brunette with medium skin, but in

> **Bet You Didn't Know . . .**
> Animals can make their own vitamin C. It's made in their livers from a simple sugar called glucose.
>
> Unfortunately, we *Homo sapiens* can't manufacture our own stores of C; our livers lack the enzyme that would make this possible. So if we do not add lots of C to our diets, we quickly become deficient, which can lead to a host of health problems.

my 42 years I've spent a lot of time in the sun without protecting my skin," Patricia told me. "I wasn't ready for cosmetic surgery, but I was uncomfortable with the laugh lines that were starting to form around my nose and the crinkles on my upper lip."

Patricia didn't think any treatment would help her sun-damaged skin — including vitamin C ester, which she first used in one of my clinical trials.

"All I did was apply the vitamin C ester cream to my face twice a day, after washing with my normal cleanser," Patricia reported. "After 30 days, I was blown away. My skin glowed. It looked . . . revitalized. My skin seemed to have tightened. And my crow's feet? Not only did they fade; some of them actually disappeared. I looked so radiant, in fact, that my mother-in-law looked

> ### When to Say "Si" to C
> All antioxidants are not created equal. But even more important, some are better suited to some skin repair jobs than they are to others. Here are the skin conditions most likely to respond to treatment with vitamin C ester topical preparations:
> - Fine lines and wrinkles on severely sun-damaged skin
> - Sagging skin that is losing its firmness because of lost or damaged collagen
> - Sunburned, inflamed, or irritated skin

at me and said, 'What's going on? You look like you're having another baby,' " Patricia recalled.

Another of my patients, Nancy, has also seen dramatic results. "Two or three years ago, I started to notice crow's-feet around my eyes and crinkle lines on my upper lip," said the 46-year-old psychiatric counselor for teens. "I used to smoke, so I know that's where they came from. But I also have fair skin, which I know is more vulnerable to sun damage. I came into Dr. Perricone's office saying, 'I need laser therapy, collagen injections — do something quick!' " Nancy said.

As it turned out, all Nancy needed was a topical antioxidant regimen that included vitamin C ester and alpha lipoic acid, another antioxidant you will read about in chapter 6 that works near miracles on aging skin.

"After two months I started to see results," Nancy reported. "The most noticeable change was the reduction in deeply embedded lines as well as fine lines. My skin seemed firmer. I hardly wear makeup now, and I've had no need for lasers or other treatments."

Chapter 6

Alpha

Lipoic Acid

Nature's Most Powerful
Antioxidant and
Anti-Inflammatory

Imagine a substance so powerful that it can swiftly and painlessly move through the human body knitting together fissures, soothing inflammation, and pumping up the immune system. Imagine that this substance performs these astonishing feats not only on the inside of the body, but also on the surface of the skin. Alpha lipoic acid is such a substance.

Alpha lipoic acid is a completely natural molecule that exists deep inside every cell in our bodies. Like vitamin C, alpha lipoic acid has been well-known to scientists for a long time; it was discovered in 1951 by researchers who found that it was an essential component of the energy-producing part of a cell. They also revealed that when additional alpha lipoic acid is made available to living cells, it quickly enters those cells and offers extensive protection from free radicals.

Since you already know that all antioxidants, to some degree, protect us from free radicals, just what makes alpha lipoic acid so special? How can it top even vitamin C in its ability to improve the appearance of the skin? Answering these questions has been the focus of my work for much of the past 10 years — as has been finding the best uses of alpha lipoic acid for improving my patients' skin problems. The results I've seen have been nothing short of thrilling.

I have not been alone in researching the potential of this amazing natural chemical. The past 10 years have been marked by intensive research into all the therapeutic benefits that alpha lipoic acid can provide, both when taken orally and when applied to the skin. In particular, Lester Packer, Ph.D., a researcher at the University of California, Berkeley, has reviewed and published many of the therapeutic benefits seen when alpha lipoic acid was administered orally to both animals and humans.

What have we learned? For one, that alpha lipoic acid can increase the positive effects of other antioxidants such as vitamins C and E. Dr. Packer proved that alpha lipoic acid actually protects these vitamins in the body and helps them to do a better job of squashing free radicals.

Another reason alpha lipoic acid is so special is simply this: it is both water- and fat-soluble. That means it's a universal antioxidant. Unlike vitamins C and E, it can fight free radicals in any part of a cell and even enter into the space between cells. Free radicals do their damage by randomly moving about like a tennis ball bouncing around in a room. They can damage any part of the cell, but they do the most damage where the cell is most crowded, just like a room with lots of furniture. Therefore, the cell plasma membrane, which is the most crowded part of the cell, receives the most damage from free radicals, even though free radicals can do damage everywhere, including the cell nucleus, where DNA is kept, and the mitochondria, the little energy furnaces within the cell. Of course, the ideal situation is to protect all portions of the cell, including the plasma membrane and the essential portion of the cell.

Yet another of alpha lipoic acid's unique characteristics is its ability to affect metabolism. Since alpha lipoic acid is found naturally in the mitochondria — the parts of a cell that determine how well the cell performs its metabolic duties — it can literally affect whether the cell functions with greater or lesser speed. A higher energy level allows the cell to take in more nutrients, remove wastes, and replace damaged components. If the cell's metabolism is low, as happens when we get older, the cell does not have the energy to carry out essential functions.

Why is this important? The fact is, much like an aging person, an aging cell has a slower metabolism. Aging cells are characterized by decreased energy production, and decreased energy leads to a reduced ability to repair damage. Alpha lipoic acid can actually increase a cell's metabolism, meaning that the cell increases its energy production and capacity to heal. Alpha lipoic acid is the only known antioxidant that can do this effectively.

There's no doubt that alpha lipoic acid has an unparalleled ability to protect our overall health. But it can also work wonders on aging skin.

The Alpha Lipoic–Inflammation Connection

Just how good is alpha lipoic acid for the skin? No less than outstanding. Here are some of the hows and whys.

All the effects of alpha lipoic acid that we have just discussed in general apply not just inside the body, but to the skin as well. Alpha lipoic acid helps other antioxidants such as vitamin C, E, and glutathione hang on longer, giving skin cells extra protection. And since alpha lipoic acid is both fat- and water-soluble, it can work in each and every part of skin cells. It even protects DNA.

But there's much more. Let's begin with inflammation. By now you should be an armchair expert on the effects of inflammation on aging. Inflammation of the skin is an open invitation to lines and wrinkles. When it comes to inflammation, most antioxidants have about as much strength as they do against free radicals — they can repair and prevent damage to a limited extent.

The problem is that antioxidant protection fades quickly when a cell is overwhelmed by a large number of free radicals. Alpha lipoic acid has more staying power than other antioxidants, and, as mentioned, it has the ability to help its weaker antioxidant cousins perform more efficiently. This super-antioxidant's special skill at bashing free radicals comes, at least in part, from its ability to prevent the action of a certain transcription factor called NFk-B (known in full as *Nuclear Factor Kappa B*). Alpha lipoic acid prevents the activation of NFk-B and by doing so, prevents the cell from producing the pro-inflammatory chemicals called cytokines that damage the cell and accelerate aging. In addition, once NFk-B is activated, lipoic acid can prevent further damage by scooping up free radicals that are caused by pro-inflammatory chemicals.

In chapter 2, I explained that transcription factors are messengers that deliver signals to the cell's nucleus to begin producing all sorts of enzymes and chemicals. When transcription factors function properly, they do great work. When they are in overdrive, however, they can send the wrong types of messages and thereby trigger inflammation and free-radical damage. So when alpha lipoic acid prevents the activation of NFk-B, it is essentially putting free radicals on hold as well. The result: The damage to a cell (or a group of cells — those that make up your skin, for example) stops in seconds. No other antioxidants are as effective as alpha lipoic acid in this regard.

As previously mentioned, another transcription factor, called AP-1, can either damage or heal skin (by attacking or repairing collagen) depending on how it is activated. When AP-1 is activated by sunlight, the sun exposure can cause a proliferation of free radicals in the skin. The sunlight-activated AP-1 makes the cell produce collagen-digesting enzymes called *metaloproteinases*. This type of enzyme attacks healthy collagen and causes microscarring, which eventually becomes a wrinkle.

Conversely, powerful antioxidants such as alpha lipoic acid can also activate the transcription factor AP-1. But rather than attacking the healthy collagen, the alpha lipoic acid allows AP-1 to turn on the production of other collagen-digesting enzymes. These enzymes actually digest only the damaged collagen, resulting in the elimination and erasing of wrinkles and facial scars. The result: We see an improvement in facial lines as well as facial scars when alpha lipoic acid is applied topically.

The Sugar–Aging Connection

There is yet another way that alpha lipoic acid helps the skin, and it is related to sugar. Sugar, just like oxygen, is necessary for our cells to stay alive. Unfortunately, the sugar in our bodies — called glucose — can be toxic to our cells in many ways. Sugar is exceptionally damaging to your skin because it attaches to the proteins of collagen, causing collagen to "cross-link." When collagen cross-links, it becomes stiff and inflexible, leading to the wrinkling and stiffness of old skin.

Alpha lipoic acid is a unique antioxidant because it prevents the attachment of sugar to protein (a process known as *glycation*). Once sugar is attached to protein, these proteins are cross-linked. That is, these tiny little strands, or strings, which normally slide over one another are now attached and they cannot move freely. This results in sagging and inflexible skin that gives us the appearance of aging. Alpha lipoic acid prevents and may even reverse the attachment of sugar to collagen by allowing better metabolism of sugar in the cell, preventing its buildup and also by allowing the body's natural repair mechanisms to work better. In other words, it prevents the accelerated aging of collagen by protecting it from sugar's toxic effects. In fact, when alpha lipoic acid is taken orally, it protects all of the proteins in our body from glycation and helps cells take up sugar and use it for fuel much more efficiently. That explains why alpha lipoic acid is extremely effective when taken orally to protect us from various problems that diabetics suffer from. (It should be known that people with diabetes age one-

Case Study: Better Skin at Any Age

At age 30, Jessica's problem wasn't exactly aging so much as skin that was showing wear and tear from her lifestyle and her tendency to break out. "I'm a professional cook, and that means I spend a lot of time in a hot kitchen," Jessica explained. "On top of that, I'm always leaning over food that's grilling or frying, and it makes my skin break out."

Like many people who share Jessica's Italian and Portuguese heritage, she is blessed with naturally moist olive skin, but that also means she's prone to dark circles around the eyes.

"I had little circles and shadows under my eyes when I went to Dr. Perricone," said Jessica, a Connecticut resident. "Besides, at age 30, I wanted to start taking better care of my skin.

"Dr. Perricone gave me a cleanser and cream containing alpha lipoic acid, so I put aside my department store products and started using his products daily. The first thing I noticed was that my complexion became a lot softer, smoother, and more refined. For the first time in my life, I started getting constant compliments about how great my skin looked. Then the bags and shadows begin to fade, along with the break-

> outs on my cheeks. I've now been using the product for two years, and I've never thought about going back to my other skin care products," Jessica reported.

third faster than nondiabetic people just because of the toxic effects of sugar.) Additionally, there is some evidence that alpha lipoic acid can *reverse* glycation or the sugar damage that has already occurred, either when applied to the skin or taken internally.

Of course, when it comes to sugar toxicity, the answer isn't merely alpha lipoic acid. The real answer is to eat less sugar. The anti-inflammatory diet I outline later in this book was crafted to regulate the amount of sugar you take into your bloodstream. It will help protect you from the toxic effects of sugar and the associated accelerated aging process. As you can see, alpha lipoic acid is an unparalleled weapon in the battle against aging.

Scientists are currently looking into its ability to help with heart disease, diabetes, and even AIDS. In a recent study, Jürgen Fuchs, M.D., Ph.D., of the department of dermatology at the J. W. Goethe University Medical School in Frankfurt, Germany, found that giving alpha lipoic acid to people with HIV/AIDS actually decreased the

Case Study: Erasing Years in a Handful of Days

Working hard can wreak havoc on anyone's complexion, but Carla Mancini's career posed a unique skin care dilemma. "I own an auto body shop," said the 64-year-old Connecticut resident. "Even though I work in the office, there's just oil and dust everywhere — very fine dust from sanding. Somewhere along the way, I started to notice that in addition to getting little lines under my eyes, around my mouth, and over my lips, my pores started to get larger, and my skin had this gray appearance," Carla recalls.

"It was like the oil and dust were affecting my skin tone. So I got together with a close friend, who was also upset about her looks, and we both decided it was time for us to have face-lifts.

"Once I went to the surgeon, however, he told me I had to lose all of the weight I wanted to before he could do anything. During the months it took me to diet, I heard about Dr. Perricone and went in for a consultation.

"Just about the first thing he said to me was, 'You do not need a face-lift.' He started me on alpha lipoic acid cream, and three days later, my face started to glow," Carla said. "I kept using the products, and I can now (two years later) say that I am 64 years old and I do not have wrinkles. People tell me how great I look — even my son. It's a surprise to me, because I have classic Italian skin with big pores. I never had great skin. Oh, and I'm also on the doctor's antioxidant vitamin regimen. I just can't say enough about this treatment.

"While I was using the alpha lipoic acid, by the way, my friend went through with the face-lift. When I dropped by to see her and saw the shape she was in, my blood pressure shot up and I actually fainted. I was shocked. I was not prepared for the bruising and bandages. The face-lift was definitely not for me," Carla said.

number of immune cells that are destroyed by the virus. In these pages, we are concerned only with alpha lipoic acid's ability to rejuvenate the skin, but I'm sure we'll be hearing more about this amazing antioxidant in years to come!

From the Lab to Life

The effectiveness of orally administered alpha lipoic acid in lab tests was unquestioned by the time I began my work in 1990, but the one thing that had not been tested or proved was whether this antioxidant would truly enhance the appearance and health of skin when used as a topical treatment.

I began my research with just 15 of my patients, ages 35 to 55, who enthusiastically volunteered when I told them they would be the first to test a new anti-aging treatment. All study participants were asked to rub a solution of 1 percent alpha lipoic acid (in a lecithin-based lotion) on their faces twice a day. At first, the subjects were monitored daily to make sure that there were no adverse effects, such as irritation or allergic reaction. No side effects appeared, but some participants did see immediate benefits from the lotion. Within one or two days, under-eye puffiness decreased in several participants.

I was delighted, but not surprised. Swelling, known in the medical field as *edema,* is caused by inflammation. It is an established fact that under-eye puffiness, or edema, is the result of inflammation in this area on the face. Because of its anti-inflammatory powers, alpha lipoic acid began to solve the edema quickly. Within five days, participants began to report that their skin had a healthy glow. Again, this result was expected given alpha lipoic acid's ability to promote the healthy production of nitric oxide, which helps control the blood flow to the skin.

After approximately two weeks, I started to see a reduction in the numbers of enlarged pores among many of the study participants. This finding was a bit of a shock to me, since enlarged pores rarely, if ever, respond to even state-of-the-art skin treatments such as Retin-A or alpha hydroxy acids.

At the three-month mark, the complexions of the study participants who had the largest pores and very ruddy skin began to take on a porcelain-like appearance. How alpha lipoic acid managed to actually improve the texture of the skin in these patients is not completely understood. I hypothesized that it was connected to the antioxidant's ability to increase energy metabolism, which could normalize the secretions of these sebaceous glands, resulting in smaller pores.

Between weeks 4 and 8 of the study, I began to notice that all participants were experiencing significant reductions in the fine lines around their eyes. Between weeks 8 and 12, they exhibited a decrease in the depth of deep facial lines. The one great surprise was that scars diminished on some of my patients after they began using the lotion. I did not have an explanation, but a group of plastic surgeons is conducting double-blind, placebo-controlled studies to determine if alpha lipoic acid can prevent scarring altogether. In addition, in a subsequent study I performed in my office on acne scars, my patients experienced an overall 70 to 80 percent improvement after six months of using the topical lotion.

Some of the study participants suffered from rosacea. Rosacea is a skin problem that usually occurs in people over 35 and is characterized by redness, bumps that look very much like acne, and broken blood vessels. When a few of the participants with rosacea came in for a two-week follow-up, they were actually quite upset. I had been treating them for rosacea with a standard topical antibiotic, metronidazole, which does improve the condition. But my patients noted that the redness associated with rosacea dramatically resolved over the two weeks that they used the alpha lipoic acid cream. They were unhappy because they wanted to know why I hadn't prescribed alpha lipoic acid years ago. I had to explain to them that I really hadn't had any idea that alpha lipoic acid would work to treat rosacea. Since then, a study I conducted in my office with rosacea patients proved that alpha lipoic acid lotion applied twice daily to the face can dramatically reduce the redness associated with this condition. This finding shouldn't have been surprising to me since the redness seen in rosacea often is created or perpetuated by inflammatory medication that is applied to the skin. Alpha lipoic acid, with its powerful anti-inflammatory effect, as well as the ability to scoop up free radicals, performed as predicted.

As great as the measurable, clinical results of my study were, I was truly delighted with the attitude of the study participants. When I told them the study was over, they absolutely refused to stop using the cream! I had to continue producing the treatment to keep those 15 patients happy.

Needless to say, I was ecstatic about the study results. After years of working with antioxidants, I knew I had finally found the ultimate wrinkle cure. Alpha lipoic acid not only made other antioxidants more powerful; it proved it could do just about everything for the skin that vitamin C, alpha hydroxy acids, and other treatments could not. With these two nutrients — vitamin C ester and alpha lipoic acid — I had found a way to reduce, and in some cases eliminate, fine lines, wrinkles and furrows, sallow or

When Alpha Lipoic Acid Is Best for You

In addition to making your skin look fabulous, alpha lipoic acid is natural and non-toxic. It is perfect for people who are prone to allergic reactions to other types of skin products. It works to improve the overall appearance of the skin, but it is at its best treating these problems:
- Lines and wrinkles
- Under-eye bags and puffiness
- Enlarged pores
- Acne scars
- Sallow or dull skin

dull skin tones, and puffy or dark under-eye circles. There was only one type of skin damage I saw on a regular basis that I felt still needed more attention — the lack of firmness, especially around the jawline, that many people begin to see around age 40. So I turned back to the lab and all of the known research on aging skin to look for a way to complement the amazing work of these antioxidants. The result of my work was a nutrient complex called DMAE, which you'll hear all about in the next chapter.

As for alpha lipoic acid, it's now widely available in creams, lotions, and masks from a range and variety of dermatologists and plastic surgeons. And, like vitamin C ester products, it is available in some lines in limited distribution in department stores. (See Resources on page 262.)

Chapter 7

DMAE

An Instant Anti-Aging Face-Lift

Go ahead. Sink your teeth into a delectable chocolate-fudge brownie. Plunge into a cool stream on a hot day. Pamper yourself with a long, sensuous massage. All three experiences promise one fantastic payoff — instant gratification. A surge of pleasure and satisfaction floods your senses seconds after you indulge yourself.

You can give your skin the same kind of quick satisfaction. In just about the time it takes you to finish a sinful dessert, DMAE complex can produce a visible and gratifying improvement. If you've shied away from so-called *treatments* because the very word conjures up visions of spending days carefully applying this and dipping in that until you finally see results, DMAE will change your mind. It's quick, it's easy, and it works.

DMAE is a great little acronym that's

easier to say than the tongue twister *dimethylaminoethanol*. Mixed in a cocktail with other nutrients, combined with an antioxidant base, and applied topically, DMAE can quickly and dramatically improve the appearance of sagging skin. As an added bonus, DMAE boosts the effects of other antioxidants, resulting in increased smoothness, brightness, and line reduction.

What, exactly, is DMAE? Unlike the antioxidants I've discussed so far, DMAE is an antioxidant membrane stabilizer. Because of its unique structure, DMAE actually intersperses and becomes part of the cell plasma membrane. When this occurs, the membrane is more able to resist stress and therefore is stabilized. DMAE also gives some protection from free radicals — probably by preventing the other portions of the cell membrane from being attacked by free radicals — and therefore can act as an antioxidant. Thus, DMAE is an antioxidant membrane stabilizer. It prevents breakdown of the cell plasma membrane and the resulting production of arachidonic acid and a bunch of pro-inflammatory mediators. When mixed with other amino acids and nutrients, it has a dramatic firming effect on skin.

Why Your Skin Goes South

Before we look into how DMAE firms the skin, it is important to understand why skin sags as we get older. Aging, particularly of the face, is characterized by many changes in the skin, including wrinkling, discoloration, mottling, broken blood vessels, and a decrease in radiance. But the face doesn't show age just because of changes to the skin's surface. Another very significant factor is the loss of firmness. When the skin under the chin and on the nose and the jowls begins to fall, lots of people yell "face-lift!" and run to the nearest plastic surgeon. That response makes sense given that we've all been taught that surgery is the only way to address sagging skin.

The skin itself does not actually come loose from its moorings and give in to the force of gravity. There's more to the process than that. As we age, the chemicals and nutritional precursors that give muscles that hold the skin maximum tone start to diminish as a result of years of free-radical damage. When a plastic surgeon performs a procedure designed to tighten the skin, he does not really focus on the skin itself as much as on the muscles underneath. He works deep below the skin's surface, pulling those muscles back into place, suturing them so that they will heal in a new position. The overall effect is a more youthful look, because the muscles appear to have suddenly recovered their tone.

Why do muscles sag? It helps to know a little bit about the physiology and chemistry of muscles and skin. When you move a muscle in your arm, or contract the muscles of your face to smile, a signal travels along a nerve (which functions very much like an electrical wire) to the muscle that has been pressed into service. At the very tip of the nerve ending is a bulb, which serves as a reservoir for chemicals, among them acetylcholine.

The nerve — or wire — does not directly connect with the muscle. It stops a short distance before the point of contact. At this junction, a series of chemicals is released, including acetylcholine, that causes the muscle to contract. When the nerve wants to tell the muscle that it's time to get to work, the bulb at the nerve ending gives the muscle a quick shot of acetylcholine, as a sort of neuromuscular wake-up call. Whenever the proper amount of acetylcholine is delivered to the muscle tissue, it responds with baseline muscle tone or movement.

Like all the systems in the body, the nervous system ages as a result of continued free radical damage and less than optimum nutrition. Once aging begins, the amount of acetylcholine produced, as well as the effect of the chemical on the muscle, is diminished. The only way to reverse the process — producing a stronger muscle contraction and firmer skin — is to actually increase the levels of active acetylcholine in the body. That can be achieved by improving your eating habits and using DMAE both internally and externally. The results will be better general health and an optimal nutritional environment for the skin.

How DMAE Helps

One of the best places to find DMAE is in fish — nature's brain food. DMAE will increase the chemicals in the central nervous system that help us to think clearly. Millions of people take DMAE capsules simply to increase cognitive function.

Although DMAE has a very impressive record as a successful defense against aging, it is not traditionally thought of as an antioxidant. Conventional thinking aside, however, DMAE acts as an antioxidant because it helps stabilize cell membranes, protecting them from free-radical damage by helping cells to expel waste and hold on to valuable nutrients.

When this unusual nutrient complex is applied topically, not only does it work quickly — within minutes of application; it also continues to firm the skin over time. And it couldn't be safer. It's considered a food-grade substance, so you could actually eat it without doing yourself any harm, although I don't recommend that you try.

Soothing Super-Stressed Skin

Study after study has pointed out the effects of stress on health, but a few studies have also made note of the fact that living life on the high wire can take its toll on your looks. Martha, a 41-year-old college administrator from Connecticut, learned the hard way what stress could do to her lovely Irish complexion.

"I had a very stressful job," Martha said, "and slowly but surely I started to see lines forming around my eyes, brow, and mouth. Some were frown lines, and I guess others were expression lines, but they definitely became noticeable because of my job.

"I heard about Dr. Perricone's work, so I went in for a consultation, and he gave me a treatment with alpha lipoic acid, and vitamin C ester containing DMAE. After using it for a brief time, it took a lot of the stress right off my face," Martha reported. "I was also losing tone under my chin, and my skin tightened right up after I started using the treatment.

"Overall, the lines on my face softened, and my skin got sort of a glow. But one of the things I liked best was that the treatments feel good on my skin. They're not at all heavy," Martha said.

Putting DMAE to the Test

When I put DMAE to the test as part of a clinical study, I could clearly see a difference. Experimenting with 17 selected patients, I applied the DMAE lotion to half the face and neck of each patient and then waited 20 to 30 minutes. A dermatologist and cosmetic expert were then asked if they could tell the difference between the treated and untreated sides of the faces. The improvement in the treated skin could be seen clearly. The treated sides showed an increase in skin tone, producing tighter, more youthful-looking faces. The effect lasted for approximately 24 hours.

Later I determined that long-term use of DMAE could help to permanently increase the firmness of the skin. When I tested DMAE lotion on my patients for long periods of time, my patients and I saw incredible results. The first thing my patients reported was that they achieved a leaner look because the muscle tone in their faces improved. One female patient in her forties told me that several people she met asked what kind of diet she had been on. They thought she had lost thirty pounds. Her photographs told the same story: her face definitely looked firmer and more defined.

With prolonged use, some patients have even noticed that the tip of their noses got a bit of a lift owing to the increased muscle tone that DMAE brought about in their foreheads. Believe me, there is nothing that gives a face a more youthful look than raising the sagging tip of the nose.

Several study subjects brought another finding to my attention: their noses actually seemed thinner after repeated use of the DMAE lotion. One of the most exciting changes, however, occurred when we measured DMAE's effects on study participants' necks and jawlines. After only one application of the treatment, skin tone in the neck visibly improved. Within a few weeks of use, the jawline became more defined.

Their Faces Are Her Fortune

When it comes to making the "beautiful people," well, beautiful, no one does it better than Maria Verel, celebrity makeup artist. Maria has created classic, glamorous looks, hallmarked by dewy, healthy-looking skin, for a list of notables that includes award-winning TV anchor/journalist Diane Sawyer; Grammy nominee jazz artist Diana Krall; the legendary Grammy Award–winning singer Emmylou Harris; Hollywood mogul and author Nora Ephron; hit fashion designer Cynthia Rowley; Emme, host of E! Entertainment Television's *Fashion Emergency*; and the actress Michael Michele.

"My goal is to ensure that each individual radiates his or her own beauty and doesn't look made up." And Maria has a secret (or she did until now): She incorporates NVPerricone Cosmeceuticals containing alpha lipoic acid and DMAE complex into her color cosmetics. Most often she applies them directly to bare skin before considering a stroke of color or contrast. "When I use Dr. Perricone's alpha lipoic acid and DMAE preparations under makeup, it makes skin glow," Maria continues.

"My clients are often subjected to grueling schedules, yet they still are expected to look great all the time. They want to look fabulous but not artificial," Maria explains. "I audition every available product on the market; my makeup case holds the range from La Prairie and Chanel to Oil of Olay and Neutrogena, and NVPerricone antioxidant products really stand apart.

"Dr. Perricone brings science to the art of beauty. These are truly the most exciting skin products I've ever seen and a cornerstone for me in perfecting my art. The extraordinary benefits of NVPerricone products ensure that I will be using them for many years to come, both personally and professionally."

The most dramatic effect, however, was the natural lift that DMAE produced in the eyelids. All study participants reported a tighter, more toned appearance in the skin around the eyes after just a few days of use.

Fuller, Firmer Lips

DMAE, combined with antioxidants, can also help with another beauty dilemma — thin or aging skin around the lips. In the right combination, this compound can actually plump up lips that are too thin or are showing fine lines and wrinkles. Perhaps the best description of how this combination works comes from professional makeup artist Matthew Van Leeuwen. In a recent issue of *In Style* magazine, he said that he never applies lip color to any of his clients unless he prepares their lips with DMAE complex (as a lip plumper) first. "It makes lips look as if you just made out for half an hour," Van Leeuwen says.

Is he imagining things? Not at all. Clinical studies show that DMAE actually helps increase circulation and tone to the lips, creating a fuller, firmer appearance.

A Bonanza for Your Body, Too

Perhaps best of all, the affects of the DMAE treatments do not stop with the face and neck. I've conducted another study to measure the effects of a DMAE lotion, slightly stronger than the solution used on the face, on the back of the legs and buttocks. When the lotion was applied to this area, a visible improvement in dimpling was seen within 20 minutes. The body toning lotion even produced noticeable results in study participants as young as their twenties. Much to my surprise, DMAE body lotion has developed quite a following among bodybuilders who use it before they

What DMAE Does Best

DMAE is a booster that enhances the strength of other antioxidant therapies. Look for this skin care ingredient if your problem is:

- Loss of firmness in the skin on the face or body
- Fine lines above and below the lips
- Stressed, overtired skin
- Thin lips that you want to look fuller and more defined

DMAE preparations are typically available at cosmetics counters in better department stores; check the Resources (page 262) for further information about where to obtain them. Types and frequency of application vary by product, so be sure to read labels carefully before using.

appear in competitions! They say it helps them show more muscle definition.

One of the best uses for a DMAE body lotion, however, is on those occasions when you want to look your absolute best in an evening gown, bathing suit, or any other outfit that's a little revealing. It's guaranteed to give you a beautiful, smooth, firm look — even after just one application. It is no surprise that many people who depend on their looks to make their living have made DMAE complex a regular part of their makeup and grooming regimen.

If you combine alpha lipoic acid and vitamin C ester containing DMAE, you can address every sign of aging, and significantly, if not completely, remove the lines, wrinkles, discolorations, and loss of firmness that are inevitable. The changes associated with aging are unavoidable, but they can all be successfully treated, with few or no side effects, allergic reactions, invasive procedures, or pain.

But even these incredible antioxidants are only part of what science has to offer in the very near future. The antioxidant revolution has just begun. New and better natural ways to repair, rejuvenate, and protect your skin are, no doubt, well on their way.

Chapter 8

Undercover Antioxidants

Alpha Hydroxy and Beta Hydroxy Acids

If there were a book titled *Great Moments in Skin Care*, at least one chapter would have to be dedicated to alpha and beta hydroxy acids — the acids of the 1980s. Way back then, before you probably even thought about wrinkles or laugh lines, hydroxy acids were the first skin care ingredients to bring the whole concept of skin treatments to a new level. They had been around forever, in one guise or another, but it wasn't until the 1980s that scientists finally figured out how to concentrate them in creams and lotions. These master exfoliants (as they were thought of at the time) were a giant step beyond moisturizers, and they made a visible difference in the skin. Fast-forward to the year 2000, and antioxidants are definitely taking center stage, but with one, well-kept secret: the hydroxys are still part of the team.

Even my fellow dermatologists wanted to

know why I would be including a chapter on alpha and beta hydroxy acids in a book about antioxidants. The answer is that the hydroxy acids are antioxidants too! Alpha hydroxy is a designation for a group of acids that are derived from foods. Glycolic acid, one of the most popular alpha hydroxy acids, is derived from sugarcane, and lactic acid is derived from milk. When applied to our skin, glycolic acid helps to exfoliate, that is, take off the dead cells, giving us a younger appearance. What's more, alpha and beta hydroxy acids are a valuable addition to many of the new super-antioxidant products (such as alpha lipoic acid containing DMAE complex, for example) because they work synergistically with other antioxidants, enhancing their antioxidant activity.

An Ancient Beauty Secret

In case you haven't heard by now, Cleopatra beat everybody to the punch when she figured out that alpha hydroxy acids could add a certain glow to her legendary skin. Thousands of years ago her highness was famous for her milk baths. Milk is packed with lactic acid, one of the most effective alpha hydroxies of them all. By the late 19th and early 20th centuries, Scandinavians were using them as well. In 1976 E. J. Van Scott, M.D. and R. J. Yu, Ph.D., reported on the efficacy of glycolic acid in treating a disease characterized by scaling skin called *ichthyosis*. But it was not until the early 1990s that major cosmetics companies recognized the potential of alpha and beta hydroxy acids as additives to skin creams, lotions, and cleansers.

Hydroxies in Medicine

In 1982 while I was still an intern at the Yale School of Medicine (in pediatrics, my first medical concentration, before I chose dermatology), and long before I ever read about the topical uses of glycolic acid, I became interested in a disease that was all too common among African-American patients at Yale-New Haven hospital — sickle-cell anemia. This disease is characterized by acute episodes of severe pain and fever, which can lead to death. The problem is that a single amino acid is substituted in the beta chain of the hemoglobin molecule, which causes the hemoglobin to polymerize (form a compound) when there is reduced oxygen within the molecule. The result is a physical deformation of the red blood cells.

When seen under the microscope, these red blood cells look like sickles instead of round donuts, the normal shape of red blood cells. The sickle-shaped red blood cell clogs the small arteries, resulting in severe pain and dysfunction in many organs such as the spleen.

It is important to note that the red blood cells in these patients do not sickle when oxygen is present in the cell. The sickling process occurs only after the cell has given up its oxygen to the tissue. The question asked back then, of course, was how could this information be used to help sickle-cell patients? I thought if we could find a way for the red blood cells to hold on to oxygen rather than give it up, we could prevent sickling. I found that glycolic acid, an alpha hydroxy acid, could accomplish this task, at least in a test tube. So hydroxy acids have been found to be effective not just in skin care; they also have the potential to help with serious, debilitating diseases.

When my pediatric internship came to an end and I moved on to my dermatology residency, I discovered more research on glycolic acid. In addition, during this period, in 1985, I was actively working with topical vitamin C as a treatment for free-radical damage to the skin. One day, while looking at drawings of the molecular structure of both substances, I noticed that portions of the glycolic acid molecule bore a marked similarity to a portion of the vitamin C molecule. Since I had already experienced the antioxidant powers of vitamin C, I immediately became interested in focusing on glycolic acid in my clinical studies. I hypothesized that since the structures of vitamin C and glycolic acid were so similar, perhaps glycolic acid functions similarly to vitamin C. In order to test this theory, I applied glycolic acid lotion to patients who had been sunburned, and it appeared as if it was reducing the redness more quickly than if the skin went untreated. I considered that the glycolic molecule could very well act as an antioxidant, thereby providing protection against free-radical damage.

Since it was well-known that glycolic acid, when added to creams or lotions, helped to relieve dry skin, I began to add it to other topical treatments for my patients who were suffering from skin disorders. I found that this ingredient enhanced the penetration of many skin care treatment ingredients and therefore enhanced their effectiveness. Over time I began to recognize glycolic acid as an ideal treatment for

The Solution for Razor Bumps

Many men with brown skin find themselves plagued by ingrown hairs and razor bumps, especially after shaving. It is estimated that approximately 60 percent of black men have a condition called *pseudofolliculitis barbae* — a very fancy term used to explain the inflammation that occurs when curly hairs work their way back into the skin and produce shaving bumps.

Just about any man with skin that has a significant melanin content is at risk for developing razor bumps. A young man named Joe arrived at my office deeply concerned about the dark spots, redness, and irritation that had developed all over his face and neck as a result of shaving. He had already been seen by a dermatologist who had given him the traditional medication for the condition, which is Retin-A.

As a result of my own research, I knew that Retin-A had little effect on razor bumps, and since it can produce inflammation in some skin types, Retin-A tends to further irritate the skin around the bumps.

I had conducted a small, double-blind, placebo-controlled study with my patients and found that the best solution for razor bumps was alpha hydroxy acids. The men in my test group experienced a 60 percent reduction in the bumps caused by ingrown hairs over the course of four weeks. In addition, I discovered that if they used a glycolic acid cream, these men could shave daily without any further problems. Alpha hydroxy acids are acidic substances, most often derived from foods, that have been used for years to enhance the appearance of the skin. Lactic acid, the acid in milk, for example, is an alpha hydroxy acid. There are many creams containing alpha hydroxy acids on the market. These gentle acids help the skin to eliminate dead surface cells and heal inflammation.

So I prescribed a regimen of alpha hydroxy acid lotion twice daily for Joe, as well as a topical alpha lipoic acid solution to calm the inflamed skin on his face and neck. Over a period of eight weeks he reported that he could shave more comfortably and that many of his dark spots had disappeared. He was also delighted to find that the few fine lines he had accumulated in his 36 years had faded, along with his razor bumps.

people with serious skin problems — such as dermatitis or razor bumps. But gradually I noticed that patients treated with glycolic acid lotions also enjoyed a reduction in fine lines and brown, pigmented areas (most often called *age* spots).

As I entered my third year of residency in dermatology, I had the opportunity to meet with Dr. Van Scott, who had published the original papers in 1976 on the efficacy of glycolic acid to treat scaling skin disorders. I told him how effective alpha hydroxy acids appeared to be in the treatment of aging skin. I thought the time was right to ask cosmetic companies if they were ready to work with alpha hydroxy acids. Much to my surprise, not a single company was interested. One company even conducted a short study to test the efficacy of glycolic acid in the treatment of dry skin and told me, in no uncertain terms, that glycolic acid was not the least bit effective. I must admit I was truly surprised by the close-minded attitude of the research and development groups at some of the larger companies. It would be several years before they woke up to the benefits of alpha hydroxy acids.

I continued to work with alpha hydroxies, however, because I was convinced they could repair damaged skin. My next discovery was that glycolic acid could relieve erythema (redness) caused by ultraviolet radiation. My studies offered proof that glycolic acid acted as an antioxidant. Not only did it ease the redness that appeared after UVA exposure, it prevented free-radical damage — in this case even better than vitamin C did.

Within seven years of my initial efforts to get cosmetic companies to take a more serious look at alpha hydroxy acids, the first product lines featuring the fruit acids began to appear.

Of course, scientists now agree that alpha hydroxy acids certainly have the ability to dramatically improve the appearance of aging skin. In addition, the use of alpha hydroxy acids in cosmetic products has become a multibillion-dollar industry. Some evidence now points to the notion that glycolic acid can stimulate collagen production very much as vitamin C does. I use glycolic acid in the antioxidant skin care formulas I prescribe for my patients. It enhances the penetration of vitamin C ester and alpha lipoic acid, while improving skin exfoliation and smoothness.

The Alphas and Betas of 2000

Now that alpha hydroxy acids are actually old news in the cosmetics marketplace, consumers are also reaping the benefits of beta hydroxy acids. The name that's most likely

> ## When Alphas and Betas Work Best
> The hydroxy acids are an important part of multiple antioxidant therapies, because they help make other products far more effective and offer a few unique benefits for aging skin, helping to treat:
> - Razor bumps
> - Rough, dry, or finely lined skin
> - Uneven pigmentation (age spots)

to sound familiar to you is salicylic acid (which is not exactly a beta hydroxy acid, but it's been commonly identified as such for so long that it has become accepted as one). Salicylic acid has been used for many years as a peeling agent for skin; that is why you'll find it included in lots of astringents, cleansers, and creams that are meant to treat dry skin conditions or acne.

Research dermatologists now believe that salicylic acid is also beneficial in the treatment of aging skin. Salicylic acid (which is related to aspirin) is an anti-inflammatory. Since the goal is to stop inflammation when one is working to prevent premature aging, salicylic acid can be a very soothing skin treatment. Many dermatologists say that this particular acid is not an antioxidant, but that's simply not the case. Not only does it scoop up highly dangerous free radicals; it has a particular affinity for one type of particularly damaging free radical called the *hydroxyl radical*. When salicylic acid picks up a hydroxyl radical, the chemical structure of the salicylic acid actually changes. Because of this process, scientists often use salicylic acid to measure free-radical activity in a test tube. In fact, salicylic acid is called a chemical trap for free radicals (a concept similar to spin traps, which you will learn all about in chapter 12). Some very preliminary studies, using small numbers of patients, seem to confirm some of these early reports. I believe that salicylic acid will take a prominent place in developing anti-aging regimens.

You can expect to continue to see alpha and beta hydroxy acids in cosmetics used in the treatment of aging skin. And, effective over-the-counter glycolic acid treatments for razor bumps are not far behind. Alpha and beta hydroxy acids may have briefly been dismissed as yesterday's cosmetic discovery, but their antioxidant properties place them firmly in the future of skin care.

Chapter 9

Beauty from the Inside Out

The Anti-Inflammatory Diet

Don't panic! This chapter is *not* about losing weight. As a matter of fact, by the time you finish reading the next few pages, you'll no longer agonize about every calorie you consume; you'll celebrate the fact that you can fight the effects of aging with every meal. Even if you decide that you're not ready to try antioxidant-based creams or lotions, you can enjoy the benefits of increased antioxidant protection for your skin through your diet. The key is eating nutrition-packed, antioxidant-rich foods.

If you're the type of person who rushes over to the nearest department store anxious to try the latest skin-smoothing miracle cream, then it's time you started getting just as excited about your trips to the grocery store. Get started in the produce aisle. Picking and choosing is easy — just about every luscious, brightly colored fruit or veg-

Antioxidant Bounty in Eye-Catching Fruits and Vegetables

The vibrant, beautiful colors of many vegetables and fruits are Mother Nature's way of telling you that those foods are loaded with antioxidants.

If you have a vegetable or fruit that has a bright or very rich color, such as deep green leafy vegetables or bright blueberries or strawberries, that hue is a signal that the fruit or vegetable in question is packed with an antioxidant system call *polyphenols*. Scientists are just beginning to understand the importance of polyphenols, but so far, it looks as if they are capable of preventing diseases such as cancer and heart disease.

etable that draws your eye can work wonders for your skin, so try one or two new foods each week. Next stop — the fresh fish and poultry counters. Eating high-quality protein will make your skin glow and give you healthier hair than ever, since your hair is 97 percent protein and needs a protein-rich diet to grow and thrive. But forgo the red meat because it is a pro-inflammatory food. Last, stroll over to the beverage aisle and fill your cart with mineral or spring water. Water is the one thing your entire body needs to perform the metabolic processes that keep you alive and keep your skin looking clear, bright, and beautiful. The inexpensive and relatively easy process of gradually adding these powerful foods to your diet will begin to take a few years off your appearance in no time.

In the next few pages, I will show you how to make your diet one of the most important parts of your skin care regimen. You can enhance the effects of my topical antioxidant program with a nutrition plan that promotes overall health. The best diet for good health and gorgeous skin is one made up of the freshest possible fruits and vegetables, combined with low-fat sources of protein, complex carbohydrates, and clean water. Also, remember that you'll never look your absolute best unless you eat right, get plenty of rest, and get at least a moderate amount of exercise.

The Future of Healthy Eating

If you read the papers or occasionally watch TV news, then you know that doctors, nutritionists, and scientists seem to be constantly changing their opinions about what we should eat. Deciphering the conflicting reports is sometimes so confusing that you'd rather just dig into a good old cheeseburger and fries and call it a day. But before you give in and consume large amounts of simple comfort foods, let me give you a few straightforward suggestions about getting the most from what you eat.

To begin with, just about every baby boomer, and his or her parents, remembers how our trusty Food and Drug Administration (FDA) once trumpeted the idea that the four food groups were best consumed according to the rules of a neat little pyramid that basically told us to pile on the carbohydrates and take it easy on the proteins. There's no doubt that the pyramid system was a good idea, but over time lots of nutritionists and doctors came to the conclusion that the pyramid needed a new look. Years of research have proved that the best diet formula for staving off everything from the visible effects of aging to heart disease and cancer is to eat large amounts of protein, make good choices about carbohydrates, and choose fruits and vegetables rather than refined, processed foods.

The logic behind this shift in thinking comes from the study of the effects of carbohydrates on levels of insulin and sugar in the body. When you consume carbohydrates, your blood sugar begins to rise and insulin is secreted by your pancreas to keep that sugar under control. The problem is that the release of insulin pushes your cellular metabolism into a mode in which it produces inflammatory chemicals (which kick-start the aging process) and encourage your body to store fats.

This whole process is very nicely described by Barry Sears, M.D., in his book *Enter the Zone* (HarperCollins, 1995). Dr. Sears explains that insulin, in high levels, tends to create chemicals in the body that encourage inflammation. The result is not only prematurely aged skin, but also degenerative diseases such as heart disease, cancer, Alzheimer's, and many other illnesses.

The best way to be sure that your insulin levels are under control is to eat foods that are low on the glycemic index — a list that tells you what foods are more likely to cause your blood sugar to rise to unhealthy levels. Foods that are high on the index, such as potatoes, corn, and peas, will boost your blood sugar because the sugar they introduce into your system is absorbed very quickly. Your goal should be to slowly remove these foods from your diet and eat larger amounts of fruits and vegetables that are low on the glycemic index such as broccoli, grapefruit, and summer squash. (See "Getting a Better Focus on Foods" on page

Required Reading

Many of the healthy eating principals discussed in this chapter are also the basis for diet programs such as the Zone and the Mediterranean diet. Even though you may not be interested in weight loss, both of these books have great recipes for high-antioxidant meals, so add them to your bookshelf. Just increase the portion sizes if you find that you are losing weight that you don't want to lose.

Pick up *Enter the Zone*, by Barry Sears (HarperCollins, 1995), and *Optimum Health* by Stephen T. Sinatra, M.D. (Bantam Books, 1998).

148.) These foods deliver sugar to your system more slowly, because they tend to have higher fiber or (healthy) fat contents.

In addition, we now know that sugar interacts with the collagen in the body in a way that creates a phenomenon called *glycosylation.* Glycosylation — also called the *Browning reaction* — causes the cross-linking of collagen, which makes skin inflexible and prone to discolorations such as age spots (brought on by overworking the melanocytes — the cells that produce pigment in the skin). The best way to avoid the Browning reaction is to keep refined and packaged sugar in your diet to a minimum,

Getting a Better Focus on Foods

Putting together antioxidant-rich meals while avoiding foods that will send your blood sugar sky high is simple once you have an idea of what to look for. Here are a few lists to use as a guideline.

Good Carbohydrates (those low on the glycemic index)

Asparagus	Citrus fruits	Pears
Beans	Honeydew	Plums
Broccoli	melon	Spinach
Blueberries	Kiwi fruit	Most
Cabbage	Leafy greens	nonstarchy
Cantaloupe	Peaches	vegetables

Bad Carbohydrates (those high on the glycemic index)

Bananas	Corn	Papaya
Breads	Fruit juices	Pasta
Carrots	(eat whole	Potatoes
Cereals pro-	fruits)	Rice
cessed with	Mangoes	Sugar
added sugar	Pancakes	Waffles

and satisfy your sweet tooth with natural confections such as fresh fruit. You may have noticed a form of packaged sugar identified as raw sugar. Unfortunately, in my

Getting a Better Focus on Foods (continued)
Antioxidant Best Bets

Avocado (but high in fat and calories)	Dark green leafy vegetables, such as spinach and kale (lightly cooked)	squash
Bell peppers		Pineapple (but high in sugar)
Berries		Salmon (fresh, broiled or poached)
Cantaloupe/ honeydew melons	Orange-colored	Tomatoes

opinion sugar is sugar, whether it's raw or snow white. You may get a few more trace minerals when you eat raw sugars, but you are still taking in sugar that will bring on glycosylation. You're much better off getting your trace minerals from healthy foods or supplements and dropping the added sugar from your diet.

It's also important to moderate your intake of dairy products, especially whole milk, since it's high in fats and arachidonic acid. Hard cheese can be a problem as well, but low-fat cottage cheese is a good source of calcium. I also recommend low-fat milk.

But there's one type of dairy product that's a great addition to your diet and an essential part of detoxifying your system before you start your new eating plan: yogurt. Yogurt keeps the intestines healthy by introducing healthy bacteria into the bowels. Lactobacillus acidophilus (some of the live cultures found in yogurt) are considered pro-biotics because they encourage the growth of healthy bacteria in the intestinal tract.

While you are limiting the amounts of sugar and dairy products in your diet, you may also need to increase the amount of protein you eat (see "Maximize Mealtime" on page 159) — especially if you're female. Protein is absolutely essential for repairing the damage done by free radicals. A lack of adequate protein in your diet prevents cellular repair and puts you on the fast track to aging. In my practice, I have consistently noticed that people who look older than their chronological age (yet are not suffering from any known disease) invariably have a low protein intake.

Research shows that women, in particular, tend to forgo protein in favor of carbohydrates because of their unique brain chemistry. Women naturally have lower levels of serotonin (a chemical in the brain) than do men. The level of serotonin in women drops even more during the menstrual cycle. Serotonin is the feel-good neurotransmitter that makes it possible for us to experience joy, serenity, and other gifts of life. When your serotonin load falls below your comfort zone, one of the best ways to get it flowing again is to indulge in a big bowl of pasta, a hefty slice of cake, or some other high-carbohydrate fare.

Men, on the other hand, have naturally high serotonin levels, so they do not crave as many carbohydrates, and tend to have diets that consist of larger amounts of protein.

And since we're on the subject of protein, it's important to mention that eating one particular type of protein — fish — helps you take advantage of another nutrient that fights inflammation: omega-3 essential fatty acids (or EFAs). The best sources of these are salmon, mackerel, herring, anchovies, snapper, bass, bluefish, and trout.

Yes, I am suggesting that you eat fat, but I am only giving you the green light to eat certain types of fat. We've all been bombarded with information about how bad fats are, especially the ones found in fatty meats like ham, sausage, and bacon. There are good fats — the EFAs. The E in EFA stands for *essential*. That means that this fatty acid is important for our health and cannot be synthesized by our cells. These fats must be obtained from dietary sources. These EFAs are divided into different types. Two of the most important ones are omega-3 EFAs (which stop inflammation) and omega-6 EFAs (which can cause inflammation). The relationship between these two fats in the body is a little tricky. Omega-3s are best for our health, but they must exist in balance with omega-6s in order for us to reap their full benefits.

Omega-3 EFAs, which are found in fish, have the ability to dramatically reduce the body's production of inflammatory compounds. They are particularly good at targeting a chemical called leukotriene-B-4 (LTB4), which is made inside your cells out of unhealthy fatty acids — mainly omega-6 EFAs — which are most often found in animal fats.

To keep aging and poor health to a minimum, your goal is to keep your omega-6 intake low and steady. The proper sources of omega-6 are corn oils, soybean oil, safflower oil, and sunflower oil. Stay away from red meats, however, because that will only throw off your omega-6/omega-3 balance, by providing high doses of omega-6 EFAs. Increase your levels of omega-3 and keep them healthy by eating lots of fish (at least one serving a day) and many types of

Curb the Carbs

Remember, carbohydrates can basically add up to sugar unless they are the right carbohydrates — those that do not secrete insulin rapidly. Enjoy lots of fresh vegetables and fruits and avoid foods such as potatoes, pasta, candy, cake, and other sweets (see "Getting a Better Focus on Foods" on page 106).

You'll also find that keeping your blood sugar levels stable will help you fight fatigue and out-of-control food cravings. Other fringe benefits of low insulin levels include an increased ability to concentrate and think clearly, and an improved sense of well-being due to high levels of serotonin.

shellfish — the primary sources of protein in my eating plan.

Healthy Habits

Before you prepare each meal, hold up three fingers and say to yourself: "I need a protein, a good source of carbohydrates, and a small amount of unsaturated fat." Therefore, your typical meal should consist of a piece of chicken or fish, fresh vegetables and fruits, and a small source of mono-unsaturated fats such as olive oil or a few nuts such as almonds or macadamias.

Add a habit called grazing — eating four to

Calculate Your Body Mass Index

To find your body mass index (BMI), locate your height in the left column. Move across the chart (to the right) until you hit your approximate weight. Then follow that column down to the corresponding BMI number at the bottom of the chart.

Height	Weight (lb)						
4'10"	91	96	100	105	110	115	119
4'11"	94	99	104	109	114	119	124
5'0"	97	102	107	112	118	123	128
5'1"	100	106	111	116	122	127	132
5'2"	104	109	115	120	126	131	136
5'3"	107	113	118	124	130	135	141
5'4"	110	116	122	128	134	140	145
5'5"	114	120	126	132	138	144	150
5'6"	118	124	130	136	142	148	155
5'7"	121	127	134	140	146	153	159
5'8"	125	131	138	144	151	158	164
5'9"	128	135	142	149	155	162	169
5'10"	132	139	146	153	160	167	174
5'11"	136	143	150	157	165	172	179
6'0"	140	147	154	162	169	177	184
BMI	**19**	**20**	**21**	**22**	**23**	**24**	**25**

Your ideal BMI? Between 20 and 25. But each woman's ideal BMI depends, in part, on her personal health risks and age. Heart disease, breast cancer, diabetes, and arthritis may all be affected by a high BMI. On the flip side, the good news for women with large BMIs is this: You can reduce health risks significantly by losing just enough weight to drop one number from your BMI.

Height	Weight (lb)						
4'10"	124	129	134	138	143	148	153
4'11"	128	133	138	143	148	153	158
5'0"	133	138	143	148	153	158	163
5'1"	137	143	148	153	158	164	169
5'2"	142	147	153	158	164	169	174
5'3"	146	152	158	163	169	175	180
5'4"	151	157	163	169	174	180	186
5'5"	156	162	168	174	180	186	192
5'6"	161	167	173	179	186	192	198
5'7"	166	172	178	185	191	197	204
5'8"	171	177	184	190	197	203	210
5'9"	176	182	189	196	203	209	216
5'10"	181	188	195	202	207	215	222
5'11"	186	193	200	208	215	222	229
6'0"	191	199	206	213	221	228	235
BMI	**26**	**27**	**28**	**29**	**30**	**31**	**32**

five small, well-balanced meals a day — and you'll keep your insulin levels balanced. The value of eating several small to medium meals is that you never overload your body with sugars or other nutrients. Even when you're eating healthy foods, you can have too much of a good thing. If you eat a very large meal, for example, you fill your gastrointestinal track with food, which then loads your bloodstream with sugar, which makes your insulin levels spike. So it's best to eat small quantities of food throughout the day.

The quantity of food you consume should depend on your body size and lean muscle mass (see "Calculate Your Body Mass Index" on page 154). But on average a sedentary woman should get about 60 grams of protein a day, 60 to 80 grams of carbohydrates, and have a few olives or a few nuts or olive oil with each meal. A sedentary man should get approximately 80 to 90 grams of protein and an equal amount of carbohydrates and fats.

So a woman who needs 60 grams of protein can have possibly 10 to 15 grams of protein at each of her meals or snacks, four to five times a day, with 10 to 15 grams of carbohydrate and a little bit of the monounsaturated fats. If you are a larger than average person, or you exercise a great deal and have a significant amount of muscle mass, your protein requirements are higher.

Basically, non-exercising individuals need about three-quarters of a gram of protein per pound of lean body mass. Lean body mass is nothing more than your weight when all the fat on your body has been subtracted. If you have 20 percent body fat, for example, and you weigh 100 pounds, your lean body mass is 80 pounds. Your protein requirements would be based on the 80 pounds of lean body mass. When it comes to protein, you would need approximately three-quarters of a gram of protein per pound of lean body mass, or approximately 55 to 60 grams of protein a day. Lean body mass can be calculated based on the chart mentioned above.

The Meal Plan

It's not necessary to adhere to a strict diet plan that dictates calorie counts for each meal in order to reap the benefits of the super-antioxidant diet. The best approach is to refer to the food categories listed below, find the amounts that are suitable for you, and use the suggested meals to begin adding antioxidant-rich choices to your daily menus, replacing unhealthy foods. As you put together your menus, remember: broil, steam, grill, or sauté — never fry. Steer clear of fatty cold cuts, red meats, and hydrogenated (hard) oils and fats.

Suggested Meals

The menus that follow are intended to help you get started. Begin by adding a new meal choice to your normal diet every few days, until you have created a whole new way of eating breakfast, lunch, and dinner. Balance your diet so that you meet a small amount of your daily nutrient needs at each meal, for example, 20 grams of protein at breakfast, 20 at lunch, and, say, 25 at dinner.

Breakfast
- Egg white and fresh vegetable omelet (add mixed vegetables of your choice and cook in olive oil) or one serving of grilled salmon. Orange and honeydew slices on the side. Herb tea.
- Slow-cooked (not instant) oatmeal with fresh apples and cinnamon, or with mixed berries. Toss in your favorite fruit during the last few minutes of cooking time to preserve freshness and flavor. Herb tea.

Maximize Mealtime

Here are the amounts of each type of food you need each day, according to your gender. You should eat four to five small meals a day.

Nutrient	Amount
Protein	For women, 50 to 60 grams per day if inactive; 60 to 80 grams if active. For men, 70 to 80 grams per day if inactive; 80 to 120 grams if active or if you have high muscle mass
Carbohydrates	Lots of fresh fruits and vegetables
EFAs	1 teaspoon of olive oil at each meal or 2 or 3 olives per meal

- Grilled salmon. Sliced tomato and red (or other sweet) onion salad sprinkled with olive oil and vinegar. A small bowl of fresh, mixed berries, such as blueberries, strawberries, and raspberries. Herb tea.
- Vanilla low-fat yogurt with sliced fresh fruit (choose one or mix in cantaloupe, honeydew, berries, peaches, plums, or pears). Start off with half of a ruby red grapefruit.

The Quick Face Fix

What should you eat before a big event? Fish, fish, and more fish.

When my patients tell me they need to look absolutely fabulous for a big night, I recommend a topical dose of DMAE complex (of course) and suggest that they concentrate on eating certain foods for 48 hours before a special occasion. You can actually produce a healthier, smoother complexion with what you eat. The idea is to load up on plenty of non-insulin-promoting high-antioxidant foods, while hydrating your skin.

Here are some meal suggestions:

Breakfast
- Fresh fruit salad, with lots of berries
- Egg white omelet

Lunch/Dinner
- Hot or cold mixed vegetable medley: broccoli; green, red, and yellow bell peppers; cauliflower; and green beans. Season the vegetables with the fresh herbs of your choice. Cook with olive oil.
- 4 to 6 ounces of freshly broiled salmon
- A salad of leafy greens, with a little bit of olive oil and lemon juice

- Fresh melon such as cantaloupe or honeydew for dessert. WARNING: Do not eat your cantaloupe before your protein (fish). The protein slows the absorption of sugars from the cantaloupe into the bloodstream, so that it does not cause a spike in your blood sugar.

These foods are primarily non-insulin-promoting and rich in anti-inflammatory properties. Also drink 8 to 10 glasses of water each day.

Lunch
- Fresh grilled tuna over arugula, with sliced tomatoes, thin-sliced onions, and black olives. Tossed salad with a dressing of olive oil, red wine vinegar, and a little fresh garlic. Sliced golden delicious apples for dessert.
- Fresh lentil and vegetable soup. (This is a slowly simmered combination of garlic, lentils, some finely chopped carrot, onions, tomatoes, with about a tablespoon of olive oil, cooked in low-fat chicken broth. Add salt, pepper, fresh parsley, and other herbs of your choice to taste.) Serve with tossed baby greens, dressed with black currant oil (best found in a health or gourmet store) and a

> **Face-Saving Foods**
>
> If you are coping with any of the skin problems listed in this chart, dietary changes can help you heal from the inside out.
>
> Acne: Eat lots of foods rich in vitamin A and beta-carotene, such as melons, spinach, and broccoli. Avoid processed foods.
>
> Dry skin: Eat foods rich in Essential Fatty Acids (EFAs), such as salmon, fresh tuna, and flaxseed oil.
>
> Roseacea: Eat lots of antioxidant-rich fruits and vegetables such as broccoli, brussels sprouts, and cantaloupe.

  splash of lemon juice.
- Fresh spinach salad with thin-sliced white-meat chicken or turkey. Add strips of red pepper, slices of fresh mushroom and fresh onion. Sprinkle shelled sunflower seeds over the salad. Toss with Dijon mustard dressing.
- Low-fat cottage cheese on romaine lettuce, served with orange slices or fresh peach slices.

Dinner
- White meat chicken and cashews sautéed in olive oil with fresh garlic, soy sauce, and broccoli. Serve with a salad of watercress and sliced cucumbers, gar-

One Step at a Time	
Making dramatic dietary changes is difficult, so here are a few suggestions for gradually improving your nutrition.	

If you tend to eat . . .	**Try this instead . . .**
Bacon	Turkey bacon
Beefsteak	Salmon steak
Ice cream	Low-fat frozen yogurt
Fried fish or chicken	Bread-crumb baked fish or chicken
Hamburgers	Turkey burgers
Pasta	Spaghetti squash
Potatoes	Butternut squash
Strawberry shortcake	Hot mixed berry compote
Waffles and syrup	Slow-cooked oats with apples, cinnamon, and a few raisins

nished with grated carrot and tossed with olive oil and vinegar.

- Turkey burger (without the bun). Mix ground turkey with a small amount of very finely chopped onion and red pepper before cooking. Serve with grilled zucchini, eggplant, and onion slices. Mix fresh strawberries and blueberries for dessert. This meal is great as lunch or dinner.

- Grilled yellowfin tuna seasoned with fresh garlic and freshly ground pepper. Steamed mixed vegetables (broccoli, cauliflower, red peppers) tossed with olive oil. Fresh blackberries and raspberries for dessert.
- Roasted white-meat turkey (it's easy to buy just the breast at the grocer). Kale sautéed in garlic and olive oil. Baked apples stuffed with walnuts and sprinkled with cinnamon for dessert.
- Baked white beans with stewed tomatoes. Combine canned or frozen white beans (without added salt) with canned stewed tomatoes (made without added sugar and easy to find in your health food store) with one tablespoon of olive oil. Bake until tender. Serve with baby collard greens sautéed in olive oil with fresh garlic and sliced Vidalia onions. For dessert, fresh sliced peaches.

Snacks

Since your goal is to eat four to five small meals per day, you can meet your small-meal requirement by munching on healthy snacks. Try:

- Half a cup of fresh, unsalted nuts
- An apple, orange, or pear

- Six black and green olives plus celery sticks
- Fresh veggies, cut up finger-food style, tossed with vinegar, soy sauce, and olive oil
- Grilled shrimp (about a half-dozen large) with garlic on skewers. Dip in soy sauce.

Chapter 10

Creating an Antioxidant Safety Net

Stopping free radicals in their tracks is a full-time job that is best accomplished by an ever-ready team of antioxidants standing guard and prepared to fight to keep your cells healthy, your skin gorgeous, and your body disease-free. Since there's no way to constantly monitor free-radical activity or measure the amount of antioxidants you have on hand at any given moment, the only way to ensure that you have 24-hour protection is to control your dietary intake of antioxidants. The best way to do that, of course, is to eat the freshest fruits and vegetables several times a day. That said, we all know that life has a way of making it nearly impossible to stick to even the most carefully crafted diet plan. No matter how committed you are to improving your eating habits, there will be days when gulping down a cup of coffee and lunching on a bagel with cream cheese are the best you can do. My solution is to offer you an easy-to-follow vitamin program that will keep antioxidants working for you, when you're too busy to track down the perfect salad or prepare a healthy meal.

I also must confess that I am a true believer in vitamin therapy. I discovered that supplements were a necessary part of maintaining good health decades ago and I've been taking daily doses ever since. My patients will tell you that if they come to me for an anti-aging program, I'm more like an overprotective parent than a physician when it comes to encouraging them to take their vitamins. For each patient, I design an antioxidant-based program to address their individual needs. I take into consideration their age, activity level, gender, and even how much stress they have to endure on an average day.

Healthy men and women in their late twenties or early thirties, for example, will probably be given fewer supplements than patients in their fifties or sixties who may be coping with chronic health problems or a great deal of stress. If you doubt that you need to add vitamins and minerals to your diet, consider this: Research shows that 97 percent of Americans eat diets that do not even give them the recommended daily allowance (RDA) of vitamins and nutrients. There are also many highly effective antioxidants, such as Coenzyme Q_{10} and pycnogenol, that are not even measured in the FDA's research.

Factors other than your basic food intake also play a large role in your ability to maintain adequate levels of antioxidant protection on any given day. Stress, sun exposure, colds, weather changes — all types of things can affect how well your body works from moment to moment. Supplementing your diet can give you additional assurance that your body is receiving the nutrition it needs. "Daily Supplements" on page 188 will provide instructions for the supplement program I recommend, but first I want to tell you why I recommend these supplements.

Vitamins: Your Daily Dose

Vitamin A. This fat-soluble vitamin truly works wonders for the skin. It's so effective, in fact, that it is prescribed (as Accutane or Retin-A) to heal severe acne and other skin problems. It also protects your hair and vision, along with your respiratory and digestive systems. Vitamin A also plays a key role in the health of bones and teeth and can stimulate wound healing. In addition, some studies have shown that this antioxidant supports immune function and increases resistance to infections, some cancers, and heart disease.

I suggest that you take only small amounts of vitamin A, however, because your body stores it up and it can become toxic. Take only 5,000 IU of vitamin A daily, or take its precursor, beta carotene, which is converted to vitamin A inside the body but does not cause toxicity.

B-complex. Several vitamins are involved in creating a B-complex supplement, and each one makes a unique contribution to keeping you healthy and giving you a gorgeous complexion. B-complex vitamins are critical links in a number of enzyme-related chemical reactions that protect the skin, and your health, in different ways. At any given time, one of the B vitamins is at work in your body spurring on carbohydrate metabolism, nervous system function, fatty acid metabolism, the maturation of red blood cells, and other important processes.

All Bs are needed in your diet, but when it comes to protecting the skin, B_6 actually converts EFAs, such as gamma linoleic acid, into active chemicals in your body called *prostaglandins*. And prostaglandins do an excellent job of controlling the chemicals that cause inflammation.

In addition, B_6 helps prevent heart disease by helping your body control its levels of homocysteine — an amino acid that can damage the heart. Other research has shown that vitamins B_1, B_2, and B_{12} play a critical role in energy production. They help provide the essential enzymes for the cellular processes that produce energy in the skin's cells, and B_1 actually helps your body make use of the energy supplied by glucose.

As powerful as the Bs are, however, it's important to remember that they are water-soluble, and therefore your body's supply needs to be replenished (through diet and supplements) on a regular basis. B_6 deficiency can cause everything from anemia to heart disease, but this deficiency is most likely to be brought on by health problems rather than dietary deficiencies. But taking large amounts of B_6 (more than 50 to 100 milligrams) can lead to nerve damage. People who consume large amounts of alcohol, suffer from liver disease, or have severe, chronic diarrhea, for example, can have dangerously low levels of B_1 or B_2. B_{12} deficiencies can also lead to anemia, which is characterized by pale skin and a loss of energy. Folic acid, the B vitamin best known for helping women have healthy babies, can also be deficient in the diet, but it's easy to remedy with an 800 micrograms daily supplement.

To get the best from the Bs, take a supplement that combines them as B-complex (see "Daily Supplements" on page 188), to be sure you get a balanced amount of each nutrient in the group.

Vitamin C. As you already know from reading chapter 5, vitamin C does miraculous things for your health. Not only does it prevent free-radical damage; it helps you to produce collagen. Since vitamin C is water-soluble (your body does not store it), you have to replenish it on a daily basis. For patients under the age of 25, I recommend a minimum of 1,000 milligrams of C daily. For older patients, people who are under a lot of stress, or smokers, I recommend a higher dose. An average 50-year-old patient should take 3,000 to 5,000 milligrams of C a day. If you are increasing your vitamin C intake, it is best to add vitamin C gradually. Larger doses can cause gastrointestinal distress; if you experience any gastrointestinal discomfort, decrease your dosage until your body has adjusted, and gradually increase the vitamin C dosage over a period of days and even weeks. Be sure to divide your doses throughout the day and take them 20 to 30 minutes before meals.

I also recommend a vitamin C supplement called ascorbyl palmitate (vitamin C ester), which is fat-soluble. A dose of about 500 milligrams a day is adequate for any age group.

Vitamin E. This fat-soluble nutrient has been celebrated as a preventive for heart disease, sunburn, and possibly even breast cancer. Younger patients should take approximately 200 IU a day. Patients in their forties and fifties should take anywhere from 400 to 800 IU a day. Make sure your supplement is made up of both vitamin E tocotrienols and gamma tocopherol, because these are the forms of E that have been found to be most effective against free-radical damage. The alpha tocopherol form of vitamin E alone is really not the best choice.

New E versus Old

Alpha Tocopherol. This is the vitamin E base of cosmetic and supplement formulations available throughout the 1990s. Some formulas may also contain mixed tocopherols. Both types of E are effective emollients and antioxidants for the skin and body. These forms of E have also been shown to prevent heart disease and have a moderate cholesterol-lowering effect.

The Tocotrienols — Super Vitamin E for Your Skin

Before the first antioxidant-based skin cream ever appeared on the market, beauty-conscious women everywhere were dabbing vitamin E oil under their eyes and on patches of dry skin because it supposedly possessed the power to make fine lines disappear. Those sticky, marginally effective preparations were replaced with more sophisticated creams, but in the 1960s and early 1970s we (scientists and physicians) did not realize that we had barely scratched the surface when it came to understanding the skin-nurturing power of vitamin E.

We were soon to discover that in science, as in life, sometimes the only way to find the key to the future is to look carefully at the past. The antioxidant revolution is just beginning, but it looks as if the next wave of skin-saving supernutrients has already been discovered. The big surprise is that a vitamin that's been right under our noses for generations is leading the pack — vitamin E.

But it is not just any form of vitamin E. It is a particular type of the vitamin that holds more promise for safeguarding our health and rejuvenating aging skin than any we've seen before. Where was this type hiding? In plain sight. When scientists selected what they thought was the most useful part of the vitamin years ago, it appears they may have made a small mistake.

Taking a Second Look

Since vitamin E is in everything from baby ointment to cooking oil, it seems as simple as Vaseline. In fact, vitamin E is a very complex substance that is made up of eight different components. The two components that are of most importance for this discussion are the tocopherols (think of this as the "old" form of vitamin E) and the tocotrienols (the "newer," more effective form that will be appearing in products in the near future). When the antioxidant effects of vitamin E were first studied 20 or more years ago, scientists concluded that alpha tocopherol, one of the eight components, was the most efficient form of E for protecting lipids from being damaged by free radicals. Lipids are a diverse group of fats that exist in all living things. All lipids are needed to help the body function properly, but one type, the *phospholipids,* which are major components of our cell membranes, control the ways in which water and other substances pass through the cell membrane. The vitamin and cosmetic industries took a good look at this research and quickly began to formulate consumer skin care and supplement products containing concentrated forms of alpha tocopherol. In addition, derivatives of alpha tocopherol such as tocopherol acetate or succinate (esters of alpha tocopherol) were added to many cosmetics.

Then in the late 1980s researchers began to look at the other components of vitamin E to see what effects, if any, they might have on health. But this time they investigated the properties of tocotrienols, instead of the tocopherols. In the lab, the differences between the two components of vitamin E could be seen immediately. Vitamin E consists of a large molecular structure that is ring-shaped. Attached to the ring is a hydrocarbon tail. Researchers thought that all the antioxidant activity of the molecule was based on the composition of the ring-structured portion of the molecule. When scientists started examining other portions of the vitamin E molecule, such as the tocotrienols, once again the ring shape was identical. The difference was that the tail of the tocotrienol hydrocarbon chain had some portions that contained an electron double bond. When there is an electron double bond in a hydrocarbon, it is called unsaturated. When scientists tested the tocotrienol form of vitamin E, that is, the molecule with the unsaturated hydracarbon chain, they found that it had very significant therapeutic effects in preventing heart disease when taken orally.

It seemed that the tocotrienol vitamin E dramatically lowered cholesterol levels in the body. This was quite a surprise because the form of vitamin E that has been in most vitamin supplements for years did seem to be somewhat protective against heart disease, but it had never been proven to affect cholesterol before. But amazingly, research shows that tocotrienols, in controlled doses, are capable of inhibiting cholesterol as efficiently as synthetic cholesterol-lowering drugs, but without the side effects.

The connection seems to be the tocotrienol vitamin E's ability to affect a certain enzyme in the body. The reason scientists were able to develop cholesterol-lowering drugs in the first place was because they discovered that one of the most effective ways to slow the body's ability to make cholesterol is to inhibit the production of an enzyme called *HMG coenzyme A reductase*. Many of the cholesterol-lowering drugs on the market are HMG coenzyme-reductase A inhibitors, but they all seem to cause some type of side effects. Scientists discovered, however, that vitamin E — in the form of tocotrienols — could also inhibit the body's production of HMG coenzyme A reductase without causing any side effects at all. This research would also play a role in the therapy I would eventually suggest for my patients.

By 1990 I had read about these exciting discoveries, and I could not help but wonder if the tocotrienols would have greater antioxidant potential than alpha tocopherol when used on the skin. My skin care research was always focused on the effect that any given antioxidant could have on a cell membrane, so I put together a study testing tocotrienols in a system that behaved much like a cell membrane called a phospholipid bilayer model.

The model is structured just like a sandwich, consisting of fats attached to groups of phosphates, like the cells in your body. I worked with the model to produce free radicals from oxidative stress, the same way that they would have naturally been created in skin that was exposed to sunlight. I then assessed the damage to the phospholipid bilayer system. I also tested the old form of vitamin E, alpha tocopherol, in the phospholipid bilayer system so that I had a basis for comparison.

When I evaluated the phospholipids for free-radical damage (the best way to do this is to measure how many peroxides form in the system) the results were very surprising. Tocotrienols inhibited peroxide formation, that is, free-radical damage, much more efficiently than did alpha tocopherol, the form of vitamin E we have been using in products for over 30 years. After making careful measurements in the lab, I discovered that tocotrienols were actually 40 to 50 times more powerful than the other forms of vitamin E. My conclusion was that we actually had the ability to dramatically increase protection of the body's cell plasma membranes, and that the substance that was making it possible had been right under our noses for years!

The secret was in the chemical structure and action of the more powerful form of vitamin E: The tocotrienols have the ability to completely disperse in a cell membrane, move about at warp speed, and scoop up free radicals far more quickly than alpha tocopherols.

The next step was to figure out how to use this incredible antioxidant on the skin.

Make the Most Powerful Choice

By the time this book reaches the stores, the very first skin care products formulated with tocotrienol vitamin E should be in production. By using a special extraction process on rice bran oil and palm fruit oil, scientists have been able to produce a liquid that has a very high concentration of tocotrienols. The extract can easily be mixed into creams, lotions, shampoos, or other cosmetics.

Preliminary research shows that tocotrienol-based preparations can make hair shinier, heal redness and scaling often seen in severely dry skin, and prevent fingernails from cracking and peeling. These preparations will also probably make sunscreens more effective, while helping to fight off the inflammation caused by sunburn. In addition, tocotrienols can be added to other cosmetics, such as lipsticks, eye makeup, and foundation, to provide all-day protection for the skin.

Become a wise consumer and watch for products containing the new form of E or ask your dermatologist to help you stay on the lookout for tocotrienol-rich products, which may begin to appear early in 2000. Adding a tocotrienol supplement to your vitamin regimen is also a great idea. It will increase your protection against heart disease as well as your overall antioxidant protection from many other illnesses. When you read the labels of topical products containing vitamin E, look for the words "High Potency E or HPE." That's your guarantee that you're getting the E that is bound to change the future of skin care.

Tocotrienol. This form of E has all the properties of alpha tocopherol or a formula of mixed tocopherols, but it is 40 to 50 times stronger and more effective at repairing skin damage, protecting the heart and circulatory system, and banishing free radicals. Tocotrienols may also be called *HPE*.

Minerals

In addition to the vitamins discussed above, I recommend that you take a multi-mineral tablet each day. Not only are minerals important for your skin; they safeguard your health in a variety of ways.

Calcium. Calcium works together with magnesium to prevent osteoporosis. I usually suggest a dose of 1,000 milligrams of calcium daily to my patients for optimum health (pregnant women or postmenopausal women should determine their proper amount after consulting their physicians).

Studies show that calcium, which is the mineral that exists in the largest quantity in the body, is needed for the growth and maintenance of bones and teeth. It also helps promote normal blood clotting and makes it possible for muscles, like your heart, to contract. Unfortunately, calcium deficiencies are fairly common — especially among people who adhere to low-calorie diets that eschew dairy products. Therefore supplements are generally recommended for just about everyone over age 30. Too much calcium, however, may contribute to constipation. For calcium to be effective in the body, you also need ample amounts of vitamin D and magnesium.

Magnesium. This is another essential ingredient in building healthy bones, but it also has an important job to do independent of other minerals. It helps your muscles relax (the opposite of calcium's effects) and helps the body convert food to energy. I recommend a dose of 400 milligrams daily.

Trace minerals. These minerals, sometimes called micro minerals, are referred to in this way because they are critical to good health, but only if they are present in the body in very small quantities, as large amounts can be toxic. Here are some of the most important ones in my plan.

- *Chromium* has recently gained a stellar reputation as a fast, fat-burning supplement that can make dieting a day at the beach. These claims are still considered controversial, but this mineral has a long and venerated reputation as an insulin regulator in the body, so it naturally slows the pro-inflammatory forces that age your skin. I suggest 200 micrograms daily. If you are diabetic, consult your physician for dosage information.

- *Selenium* is a vital antioxidant required to form glutathione peroxidase, one of our most important natural antioxidant defenses. It helps to neutralize certain toxins, such as cadmium, mercury, and arsenic. It also gives a great boost to the immune system, and some research has shown that it fights heart disease and helps to prevent cancer.

    In high doses, selenium can be toxic, so it's best to stay at 200 micrograms or below, daily.

- *Zinc* does lots of valuable work in the body, such as enhancing immune system function and contributing to bone development, energy metabolism, and wound healing. Having zinc in your diet in appropriate amounts is also essential for great-looking skin, because zinc is a member of a group of enzymes that helps your body maintain its collagen supply. Without zinc, the enzymes that digest damaged collagen and allow for the development of new collagen cannot function. Zinc is also an essential part of the enzyme super oxide dimutase (SOD), which works to break down oxygen-based free radicals. In some patients this mineral will also encourage the healing of acne scars, although scientists are still not quite sure why this occurs.

Like selenium, zinc can be toxic in large doses. I recommend 15 to 30 milligrams a day.

Other Important Supplements

Acetyl L-carnitine. I strongly recommend this supplement for people who are over age 50 and struggling to repair their skin. A daily dose of 500 to 1,500 milligrams helps repair the mitochondria, the energy-producing portion of your cells. Acetyl L-carnitine is also being used to increase cognitive function in elderly people.

Alpha lipoic acid. This super antioxidant works hard to fight free-radical damage inside and outside the body. As I

Case Study: Putting the Research to Work

Cholesterol is usually a problem addressed by internists and cardiologists, so you might be surprised to discover that elevated cholesterol levels, and the treatments that are prescribed to lower them, can have a negative effect on the appearance and condition of your skin. That was the problem facing Mary, a 63-year-old patient who came into my office complaining that her skin was so painfully dry that she was itching and experiencing all sorts of discomfort.

Mary was truly disappointed by the fact that the years seemed to be adding wrinkles, mottling, and discoloration to her face, neck, and the backs of her hands. Beautiful, glowing skin had been her best feature for most of her life. In addition to the traditional signs of aging she was seeing primarily because of a lifetime of overexposure to the sun, Mary was experiencing severe dryness that made her vulnerable to irritated skin, which often looked red and scaly.

As always, my consultation began with questions about her overall health. Mary was basically in good shape, but she was battling cholesterol levels that had climbed above a safe range. Her doctor had recommended dietary changes, but nothing had really worked. Finally, he gave her a prescription for a cholesterol-lowering drug from a group of medications called *statins,* which are HMG coenzyme A reductase inhibitors. Millions of people are taking statins and seeing healthy reductions in their cholesterol levels but they are probably unaware that in addition to lowering cholesterol, these drugs also interfere with the production of chemicals commonly found in the body, called *cofactors,* and the result is subtle changes in body chemistry.

As I explained this to Mary, I told her that one of the most common side effects of statins (brought on by the inhibited production of cofactors) is increasingly dry skin, because the statins actually slow the production of oil from the sebaceous glands. In addition, statins can destroy the body's stores of nutrients like Coenzyme Q_{10}, an important antioxidant.

Like most people, Mary was aware of the benefits of vitamin E, but she had only used the alpha tocopherol-based topical treatments most often found at cosmetic counters. The solution to her problems was to introduce her to vitamin E tocotrienols and get her started on an oral and topical tocotrienol program. I had no doubt that the combination of emollient and antioxidant benefits offered by a tocotrienol-based cream, used twice a day, would quickly heal the redness and irritation in Mary's skin, while easing the dryness and smoothing the wrinkles and fine lines that were causing her so much distress.

In addition, I had a long talk with her internist about putting her on an oral tocotrienol program to see if we could wean her off statin medications by lowering her cholesterol levels with a 50 milligram tocotrienol E supplement, plus 300 milligrams a day of Coenzyme Q_{10}.

Six weeks after her initial visit, Mary came back to me for a check-up. The dryness and redness had disappeared from her complexion, so she naturally looked much younger. Some of the glow of her earlier years had returned. She also mentioned that her energy levels were much higher now that she was taking the supplements, but she was just getting started. She said she was now ready for a full-scale, anti-aging program.

mention in chapter 6, this universal antioxidant is extraordinarily powerful: It is 400 times stronger than vitamins C and E and raises the levels of these two vitamins in the body. Alpha lipoic acid can prevent inflammatory reactions in the body and slow the onset of illnesses such as Alzheimer's disease, heart disease, and arthritis.

For people struggling with diabetes, this antioxidant can also help them regulate their blood sugar. When taken orally, and used topically, alpha lipoic acid prevents the glycation (sugar damage) of protein, meaning that it prevents the attachment of sugars to collagen, which also prevents premature aging and skin damage.

So if you are 40 or older, I suggest you take at least 100 milligrams a day.

Coenzyme Q$_{10}$. Be sure to add a Coenzyme Q$_{10}$ supplement to your nutrition regimen because this antioxidant is the one that is most easily depleted (in the skin) by sun exposure or toxins. Coenzyme Q$_{10}$ is extremely important because it gets into the cell membrane and protects it from free-radical damage. It also works in the mitochondria — the energy producing portion of your cells. This antioxidant is essential for healthy skin and a healthy heart. I suggest 30 to 100 milligrams daily for most healthy people. Those suffering from cardiac illness should consult a physician for dosage information.

I-Glutamine. This is an amino acid that protects the health of your gastrointestinal tract. It improves the health of the bowel,

Daily Supplements

Nutrient	Amount	Dosage
Vitamin A	2,500–5,000 IU	With meals
B-Complex	Balanced formula	Morning
Vitamin C	1000 mg.	Divide doses
Ascorbyl Palmitate (Vitamin C Ester)	500 mg.	Morning
Vitamin E	200–400 IU 400–800 if recommended by your physician	Morning
Calcium/ Magnesium	1,000 mg./ 400mg.	Divide into two doses — one at dinner, one at bedtime
Selenium	200 mcg.	Once daily
Zinc	15 to 30 mg.	Once daily
Chromium	200 mcg.	Once daily
Acetyl L-Carnitine	500–1,500 mg.	Divide doses — breakfast and lunch
Alpha Lipoic Acid	100 mg.	Divide doses — breakfast and lunch
Coenzyme Q_{10}	30–100 mg. daily under age 40. 100 mg. daily over age 40. Consult	Divide doses — breakfast and lunch

Nutrient	Amount	Dosage
	your physician for dosages related to heart disease.	
L-Glutamine	500 mg. to 2 grams	Divide doses — breakfast and lunch
Omega-3, omega-6 oils	2:1 ratio — 2,000/1,000 mg.	Daily
Pycnogenol	50–100 mg.	Daily

NOTE: Consult your physician for specific dosages.

prevents ulcers, and slows the breakdown of muscle tissue. It also works against liver damage because it's a precursor of many of the antioxidants that protect the liver, such as glutathione. It also helps your immune system stay in good shape. It enhances the health of the skin because it increases levels of endogenous antioxidants such as glutathione. I suggest 500 milligrams to 2 grams per day.

Omega-6/Omega-3 EFAs. Both of these oils work to consistently fight inflammation in the body. Since it's difficult to eat fish every day, it's best to take EFAs in supplement form to be sure you always have ad-

The Energy-Boosting Antioxidant

Coenzyme Q_{10} is another slightly misunderstood antioxidant that has recently been discovered as a treatment for aging skin. Coenzyme Q_{10} is found in all of the cells of the body and is responsible for energy production. The tiny energy factory inside our cells is called the mitochondria. This microscopic but mighty furnace does the work of converting molecules derived from food into energy. It should be noted that Coenzyme Q_{10} is also found in other parts of the cell. It is especially concentrated in our cell membranes. This is extremely important when we consider the cell membrane hypothesis of aging, because the amount of Coenzyme Q_{10} in a cell may tell us how fast, or by what mechanisms, that cell grows old or fights damage. Our Coenzyme Q_{10} levels begin to decline at age 40 and continue to decline throughout life.

Coenzyme Q_{10} exists naturally within our cells, but it can also be synthesized from other chemicals derived from food or supplements. It is found in red meat, salmon, and nuts.

Coenzyme Q_{10} is fat-soluble and therefore concentrates in the plasma membrane, providing protection against free-radical damage, which is why it's such a powerful antioxidant. The protective presence of Coenzyme Q_{10} is important to the cell membrane, and research has shown that this molecule is quickly used up when the skin is exposed to ultraviolet radiation or other environmental insults. Therefore I believe that it makes good sense to supplement Coenzyme Q_{10} to the cells to prevent its depletion from oxidative stress.

In addition, Coenzyme Q_{10}, like alpha lipoic acid, assists in cellular metabolism. The two molecules then work in two ways in that they can provide protection from free-radical damage within the fat area of the cell plasma membrane, as well as increase energy production in the aging cell, assisting in its repair. Coenzyme Q_{10} is extremely safe in that there are no toxic effects seen in subjects taking several hundred milligrams per day orally, but large doses (more than 150 milligrams) can lower blood pressure. Coenzyme Q_{10} seems like an ideal substance to aid in the prevention and progression of aging and other disease processes, but it can also work wonders on the skin.

A German research team recently evaluated the effectiveness of a cream containing Coenzyme Q_{10} in the treatment of fine lines on the face. The six-month study showed that individuals using a cream containing

Coenzyme Q_{10} averaged a 23 percent reduction in fine lines as opposed to the placebo group using cream without added Coenzyme Q_{10}. The results of this study are not surprising, since Coenzyme Q_{10} fits all of the criteria outlined by Dr. Nagy (the membrane theory of aging) for an effective antioxidant for human cells.

1. Coenzyme Q_{10} is fat-soluble and therefore can reach the target site, the cell plasma membrane, where a great deal of free-radical damage often takes place.
2. Coenzyme Q_{10} is nontoxic.
3. Coenzyme Q_{10} has a greater affinity for the free radicals than the molecules found in the cell membrane.

equate amounts in your system. They should only be taken in a two-to-one ratio. The amount of omega-3 should always be double the amount of omega-6. I recommend 2000/1000 milligrams per day.

Pycnogenol. The last, but certainly not the least, important antioxidant on my list is a substance called *pycnogenol.* Scientists have only recently discovered how to synthesize pycnogenol from sources such as pine bark. It works to keep skin smooth by protecting your collagen. Adding 50 to 100 milligrams a day to your diet will not only enhance your looks; it will increase your protection against chronic health conditions.

Chapter 11

Beyond

Skin

Staying One Step Ahead of the Aging Process

It is a well-worn expression, but it's still true: a journey of a thousand miles begins with a single step. The equivalent also holds for our bodies: the aging process that diminishes our appearance and vitality over the years begins with damage to a single cell.

We didn't always know this. As recently as 20 years ago, doctors and scientists had no real conception of how to address all the changes associated with aging. But with the birth of a new field referred to as *anti-aging medicine,* we have discovered ways to actually assess, control, and even reverse the processes that lead to disease, wrinkles, and other problems. Antioxidant therapy, which protects the individual cells of the body, is a critical part of any anti-aging health plan.

Do you have to take good care of your body if you want to have great looking skin? Absolutely. Just about everything you do to nurture the inside of your body enhances your outward appearance as well. Taking a simple step like drinking lots of water, for example, automatically gives you brighter, clearer eyes, improves your circulation, and makes your skin more radiant. A diet rich in protein, complex carbohydrates, and essential fatty acids cuts down inflammation, lowers your blood sugar, and gives you a healthy glow. As a bonus, eating this way also improves your mood, which can also give your looks a boost.

A diet high in antioxidants such as vitamins C and E, Coenzyme Q_{10}, and alpha lipoic acid is also guaranteed to improve the health of your gums and to promote healthier teeth. Add the amino acid cysteine, and you'll also gain healthier, shinier hair and stronger nails.

As you have probably figured out by now, *The Wrinkle Cure* approach enhances your beauty by working on your total health, not just your skin. Every aspect of my program is designed to help you increase your youth, vitality, *and* overall appearance by helping you achieve optimum health. For the best possible results, however, I recommend that you begin your program by consulting an anti-aging expert (see Resources on page 262) and putting together your own, personal program. Here's a look at what you should expect, followed by three case studies that show how successful a smartly planned anti-aging regimen can be. I hope you are as excited by these stories as I am.

Medicine to Keep the Body Young

Anti-aging medicine is a unique area of research that began to develop just about 15 years ago. The most unusual thing about anti-aging medical practices is the perspective from which doctors observe the human body. Rather than giving you a basic checkup, looking for sign of disease, an anti-aging examination seeks to measure how the various systems in your body are handling the aging process.

As we grow older, our bodies become less efficient in many ways. Our skin thins, our heart becomes a little weaker, our kidneys filter wastes differently, and our hormone levels steadily decline. All of these small — and often invisible — changes slowly add up to large and highly visible changes in our skin texture and body physique, as well as our ability to resist disease and other health problems.

These changes occur at a different pace for everyone. So the best way to determine a

Anti-Aging Tests

If you want to know what to expect from your anti-aging consultation, look over the diagnostic tests below. Your doctor should begin with this list. These tests are important for men and women with the exception of the PSA test, which is for men only.

Test	What It Does
Blood count	Measures white and red blood cells and immunity
Chemistry profile	Checks liver and kidney function, albumin and iron levels
PSA	Tests for prostate cancer
DHEA	Checks DHEA (hormone) level
Somatomedin (IGF-1)	Measures growth hormone levels
Testosterone (free and total)	Measures level of hormone
Insulin	Assesses blood sugar effects
Homocysteine	Checks risk for cardiovascular disease
TCP index	Measures the amount of protection you carry against free radicals
Lipid peroxides	Measures free-radical damage to fats in the blood
Glycation index	Measures the amount of sugars attached to your body's proteins — a high index indicates accelerated aging

egimen that will keep your body youthful is to develop a profile of how each system in your body is functioning. That's where anti-aging medicine begins.

As part of a comprehensive anti-aging checkup, your doctor will run a series of tests that will tell you how well each part of your body is working. Once it is determined where you may have nutritional deficiencies or hormonal imbalances, the doctor will design a program that will put your body back on track, and recommend nutritional and dietary changes. Using information gained through years of medical research, your doctor will design a program consisting primarily of supplements — antioxidant vitamins, minerals, and other substances. Exercise will also be part of the prescription. The idea is to maintain a cellular environment in your body that is equal to that of someone who is about 28 or 30 years old.

Who needs an anti-aging checkup? Well, just about anyone over the age of 18 or 19 can benefit from advice in how to grow older gracefully, even if "older" for them means 35. People in their forties, fifties, sixties, and beyond, however, are the ones who will see the most dramatic improvements in their appearance, health, and energy after just a few weeks on a well-designed anti-aging regimen. To gain a full understanding of how this process works, here is a detailed look at anti-aging programs I created for three clients, Linda, Harry, and Carter.

Anti-Aging Consultation 1: Linda

Linda came to me very eager to learn about how anti-aging medicine could help her improve her looks and address her problems with fatigue. She was a woman who believed in doing her homework. As soon as she sat down to talk with me, she said she had actually tried to register for my international symposium on skin and aging to learn more about the subject, but she had been disappointed to find that it was closed to everyone but health care professionals.

Since I like to get a full understanding of my patients and their concerns, I asked Linda, who was about 54 at the time, why on earth she would want to sit through a conference that was intended for scientists and physicians. She replied that she was on a quest for answers to her problems. Although I still did not have a clear idea what those problems might be, I did notice that as she spoke, there was a blank expression on her face that quickly turned to worry and sadness when she began to talk about how she felt about her health and well-being.

After about ten minutes of getting-to-know-you chitchat, I asked Linda to tell me what had really brought her to my office. Since I am a dermatologist, she started out talking about her skin. She had received a lot of sun exposure in earlier years. Like many blue-eyed blondes from her generation, she had just loved the way she looked with a tan. Of course, had she known about the damages of sun exposure, she might have decided to remain happily pale, but there was little research around to inform her, or anyone else, years ago.

She had good reason for concern. As I looked at her skin, I noticed a great deal of mottling and excess pigmentation on her forehead and cheeks, as well as fine lines and wrinkles around the eyes and mouth. She also had clusters of freckles and discoloration along her neck and her arms. These are classic signs of sun damage. But before we focused on the problems with her skin I wanted to examine the problems that lay below the surface — the problems plaguing her general physical health. A thorough anti-aging consultation really begins with an examination of problems that go far beyond lines, wrinkles, and spots.

Linda then began to talk about the things that really frightened her. Her first complaint was that her feelings of generalized fatigue had become worse in the past year. She had recently gone through menopause and had seen her physician, who had placed her on estrogen replacement therapy (ERT). At first, the estrogen replacement therapy seemed to increase her energy, but then her energy suddenly declined, and she found herself feeling worse than ever. As is often the case, she was also facing a number of issues in her personal life that had left her under tremendous stress for the past year. Linda is a successful executive with a large insurance company that had recently merged with another corporation, so she had been forced to spend months shuffling from job to job, and in the process, losing a great deal of her autonomy.

She also mentioned that she had been catching colds far more often than usual. But the most troubling concern was that she was experiencing a general sense of dissatisfaction. She was feeling depressed and unhappy about her life and her physical appearance.

I started my probing by asking her about her diet. Like so many of my female patients, Linda said she was always concerned about keeping her weight down (her slim physique was a point of pride; she was about 5 feet, 6 inches tall and weighed 135 pounds).

She mentioned that in the morning she would usually have a cup of coffee and a bagel. At lunch she would have a small salad, sometimes with a little pasta. Her dinner was often low-fat frozen food. She explained that she was also taking a women's vitamin formula on a daily basis to correct her decreased energy level. She said she was also trying to exercise and had joined a health club, but because of her schedule at work, it had become difficult to exercise regularly. Even when she did manage to drag herself down to the gym, her energy levels were so low that she felt even worse after working out.

Linda also confessed that although she did her best to steer clear of candies or cakes, her weakness for chocolate was often her undoing. She figured her little chocolate binges were at least partially justified, because they managed to pump up her sagging, midday energy levels.

One of the more nagging aspects of Linda's problems was that she was having trouble remembering things. It seems that as a college student, she was at the top of her class and had an excellent memory. In fact, until recently, she had never had to use a calendar to remember events or to bring a shopping list to the store.

Armed with this information, I told Linda that I was going to begin the diagnosis by doing some laboratory analysis. I explained that blood would be drawn so that we could take a look at her red and white blood cell count. Then I would assess other things such as her levels of hormones, including thyroid, growth hormone, and DHEA. I also referred Linda to a colleague of mine who is a specialist in internal medicine for a complete physical before she returned for her next visit. This relatively quick but thorough examination was the beginning of Linda's anti-aging workup. But I already had a lot of the information I needed to understand the source of some of her health problems.

A New Supplements Regimen

When it came time for our second appointment, the first two things on the list were to improve her diet and to get her on a smart, thorough program of antioxidant and health supplements. We'll start with the latter.

Linda said she had heard a lot about antioxidants, but she still did not understand how they worked. So I gave her a brief introduction to our old friend the free radical and explained why it was so important to keep this guy under control. I explained to her that aging actually began at the cellular level, not on the surface of the skin, as many people assume, and that free radicals were responsible for causing a great deal of cell damage. I then explained that antioxidants were actually a sort of cellular rescue team, racing around behind free radicals and repairing the scars they left behind — scars that would eventually lead to thin, sagging skin, wrinkles, illness, and other problems.

Linda then wanted to know what types of chemicals were actually antioxidants. I told her there were quite a few, but that the best known ones were familiar vitamins such as C and E. I also told her that years of research had convinced us that we all need a very high level of antioxidants in order to meet all the stresses of the average day.

She was unaware that simple things, like strolling in the sunlight or lying under artificial lights in tanning booths, could activate free radicals in the skin and cause accelerated aging. And if anyone needed to understand the free-radical damage generated by sunlight, it was a blond-haired, blue-eyed, fair-skinned woman like Linda. That little extra incentive just might be enough to get her to slather on a little extra sunscreen or grab a hat on the next particularly bright day. As you remember from chapter 3, people with light skin lack the pigment melanin, and melanin is our primary protection from the sun.

After discussing free-radical damage from exterior sources, I went into detail about the ways in which free radicals affect the healthy functioning of not only the skin, but also the organs throughout our bodies, including the brain, heart, and kidneys. After our talk, Linda was convinced that a diet rich in antioxidants was extremely important, not only to help her age gracefully but also to promote general health. So she was excited about her new plan. I assured her that the components of her antioxidant program were designed to slow or even reverse the aging process.

Here is the antioxidant program I put Linda on. It is quite extensive, but for good reason, since each component contributes in its own way.

- Vitamin A, 5,000 International Units daily
- Vitamin E, 400 International Units

daily, in a natural form containing gamma tocopherol

- Vitamin C, 1,000 milligrams, twice daily
- Grape seed extract, a powerful antioxidant that is sometimes called proanthocyanidins. Grape seed extract helps protect the collagen throughout our bodies, especially in our skin.
- Coenzyme Q_{10}, an antioxidant that concentrates in the cell membranes, protecting us from free-radical damage, 30 milligrams
- Alpha lipoic acid, 50 milligrams, three times daily

All of the components of Linda's regimen were important, but in her case, the most important supplements were the Coenzyme Q_{10} (CoQ_{10}) and the alpha lipoic acid. CoQ_{10} is especially important for women, because they have lower levels of CoQ_{10} in their bodies, and if they are eating too little protein, as Linda was, their CoQ_{10} deficiencies may be quite extreme. CoQ_{10} is essential for proper functioning of the heart, and preventing heart disease is very important for postmenopausal women. CoQ_{10} is an excellent supplement that should be taken on a regular basis by anyone interested in an anti-aging regimen.

As for the alpha lipoic acid, not only is it the best antioxidant for preventing free-radical damage in the body, it is also proven to help prevent the onset of cognitive loss. Since one of Linda's complaints was loss of memory, alpha lipoic acid was particularly important to her.

There were more supplements that I recommended. Here they are, along with explanations of their value to our health:

- Calcium, 1,000 milligrams daily, and magnesium, 500 milligrams daily. Postmenopausal women are particularly susceptible to decreased bone density, and it is now known that supplements of calcium and magnesium, as well exercise, tend to reverse bone depletion.
- Zinc, 15 milligrams daily, and selenium, 200 micrograms daily. Both of these minerals are important for the production of enzymes that help prevent free-radical damage.
- Acetyl L-carnitine, 1,000 milligrams daily. This supplement is a bit expensive, but it is worth every penny. Acetyl L-carnitine can help repair the mitochondria, the little furnaces in our cells that produce energy. This is beneficial to the appearance of our skin, as well as to

our hearts and bodies. In addition, acetyl L-carnitine has been shown to be extremely helpful in helping people with some memory loss.

- B_1 (thiamin), 20 milligrams daily
- B_2 (riboflavin), 10 milligrams daily
- B_3 (niacin amide), 20 milligrams daily
- B_5 (pantothenic acid), 250 milligrams, twice daily
- B_6 (also called paradoxine), 25 milligrams daily
- B_{12}, 500 micrograms daily
- Folic acid, 500 micrograms daily. This mix of B vitamins is important to give people the energy they need.
- Chromium, 100 micrograms daily. This mineral aids in sugar metabolism.
- Ginkgo biloba, 80 milligrams twice daily, the final recommendation. This herbal extract tends to increase circulation to the brain and can increase memory.

Next, the Eating Plan

After hearing Linda describe her eating habits, it was obvious that she was severely deficient in protein. She was getting as little as 15 to 20 grams of protein per day. This is not uncommon among women who really do not care for protein and would much rather reach for carbohydrates. This habit also made sense in light of the fact that she was under a great deal of stress and also felt somewhat depressed. Carbohydrates are one of Mother Nature's natural antidepressants because, among other things, they help raise serotonin levels.

Serotonin is a chemical in the brain — a neurotransmitter — that regulates certain behaviors and emotions. When your serotonin levels drop, you feel depressed. Women normally have lower levels of serotonin in their brains than men, and, therefore, they tend to select foods that will raise these levels, such as carbohydrates.

In addition to a very poor protein intake, Linda was also not eating enough fresh vegetables and fruits and therefore was not getting the proper amounts of vitamins, minerals, and antioxidants from her diet.

I outlined a diet for Linda that consisted of approximately 60 grams of high-quality protein a day. I gave her the following diet plan as an example of what a day's worth of food should look like for her.

- Breakfast: two scrambled egg whites, and a 2-ounce serving of non-instant oatmeal, as well as some fresh strawberries

- Lunch: approximately 4 ounces of fish, and a fresh salad with red bell pepper, tomatoes, onions, and olive oil dressing. I was particularly emphatic about the importance of salmon for her health and well-being. Salmon is rich in the essential fatty acids that are anti-inflammatory, and it is also high in protein.
- Dinner: broiled chicken with fresh broccoli, as well as garbanzo beans
- Late snack: low-fat cottage cheese and an apple

After giving her an example of an ideal day's food intake, I sat down with Linda to discuss why this was such a good meal plan for her.

Protein, which comes primarily from animal sources, is also found in some vegetables; but these proteins usually are not complete, meaning they do not have a complete profile of all the essential amino acids needed by the body to build and repair cells. Vegetarians can function well by taking in various vegetables that together have a complete amino acid profile. But I do not recommend vegetarianism for any of my patients, because I feel that the vegetarians I have treated tend to age more quickly than

Linda's Food List

Here is the list of food I recommended that Linda eat for maximum health and appearance:

Proteins

- Fish: salmon, cod, haddock, halibut, snapper, tuna
- Meat and poultry: turkey, chicken, occasional lean beef, pork, lean ham
- Vegetarian sources: soy products
- Other sources: egg whites, low-fat cottage cheese, low-fat milk, yogurt

Carbohydrates

- Vegetables: squash, spinach, onions, green beans, asparagus, cabbage, cauliflower, eggplant, collard greens, escarole, green peppers
- Fruits: strawberries, raspberries, apples, blackberries, blueberries, cantaloupe, honeydew melon, kiwi

Recommended Fats

- Olive oil, walnut oil, safflower oil, soybean oil, canola oil, sunflower oil, nut butters, avocado

Foods to Avoid

- White rice, popcorn, pasta, pancakes, carrots (raw or cooked), potatoes (especially French fries), corn (elevates blood sugar), peas the nonvegetarians. This may sound like a contradictory statement, since vegetarians eat foods with high levels of antioxidants and enzymes and also are not eating much saturated fat. But without adequate high-quality protein, the cells are unable to repair themselves as efficiently as they should. Protein is also essential to the immune system. Those people who have inadequate protein levels have more incidences of infection. Linda was fascinated to learn that an increase in protein in her diet might actually help her fight off all the colds she had been getting lately.

Next we discussed carbohydrates. Carbohydrates, which are the primary fuel of the body, come mainly from plant sources and are found in all grains, pastas, breads, vegetables, and fruits. Of course, carbohydrates fall into a couple of categories. Refined carbohydrates, which include cakes, candy, and pasta, are easily broken down by the body into glucose. Complex carbohydrates, such as whole grains and vegetables, are broken down more slowly by the body.

The distinction between refined or simple carbohydrates and complex ones is very important. If the carbohydrates we eat break down very quickly, our blood sugar rises, and this causes us to release the hormone insulin. Insulin, in large quantities, is very unhealthy, because it signals the body to store fat, increases inflammation throughout the body, and boosts the risk of heart disease. It is important that we have carbohydrates with each meal so our bodies have fuel for energy, but we should eat complex carbohydrates so as to prevent a rise in blood sugar or an insulin response.

We turned our conversation then to fat. Every diet needs some. But the worst thing we can do for our bodies and brain is to eat the wrong kind of fat: hydrogenated or partially hydrogenated oils. These are the vegetable oils that are solid at room temperature. These fats are added to many refined foods to increase flavor and consistency. They are pro-inflammatory and tend to accelerate the aging process by increasing free-radical activity. Large amounts of animal fat can have the same effect.

The other side of the spectrum — that is, the best fats — are "essential fatty acids," which can be found in olive oil, flaxseed oil, and the oils that are present in foods such as fish, avocado, almonds, and macadamia nuts. These oils help cell membranes, especially the cells of the brain. The message I gave Linda was that despite being dense in calories, fats are important to a well-rounded diet, particularly the healthy forms of fat. But at the same time, a high-fat diet can lead to increased inflammation and obesity, as well as increased risk for many diseases, such as cancer.

Once we covered all the types of food, we moved on to the frequency and amount of food Linda should be eating. I suggested that Linda eat frequent, small meals rather than just one or two large meals, because large meals tend to increase insulin production. I always recommend that my patients eat their protein first, their fruits and vegetables second, and that they avoid the refined carbohydrates entirely. Finally, I always tell them to use olive oil with their meals, since it is an excellent source of essential fatty acids.

It was also important for Linda to consume the correct quantities of food for her body size at each meal: approximately 4 ounces of protein with an equal amount of carbohydrates from the right groups, and some essential oils, such as olive oil or nuts or avocado.

Putting the Focus on Skin

Linda was the consummate cosmetics junkie. Every time she picked up a magazine and discovered a new cream, gel, or lotion promising miracles, at the very least, she rushed to the nearest department store and picked up a jar. Unfortunately, she had collected a medicine cabinet full of products that did not necessarily work for her. Many of them caused such severe skin irritations that she couldn't even use them on a daily basis.

Still, she would gallantly press forward, alternating between slightly irritating and more mild products, hoping that the benefits of the treatments would outweigh the discomfort of the irritation. Linda's at-home skin care arsenal included alpha hydroxy acids, beta hydroxy acids, retinols, toners, a myriad of moisturizers, and a topical vitamin C product that had been recommended by a friend.

I explained to Linda that anything that causes irritation to the skin kick-starts the aging process. Linda needed to understand that inflammation gives free radicals an open invitation to damage the skin. Needless to say, I asked Linda to put her current regimen on hold and try the antioxidant products that I recommended. She agreed, and we were on our way to the next step of her anti-aging solution — a new skin care program.

Since her face had a startling amount of

sun damage, I suggested that the basis of her skin care regime be topical alpha lipoic acid. Linda, ever the inquisitive patient, wanted to know where alpha lipoic acid came from. She was shocked when I explained that it was derived from potatoes. As a matter of fact, she was not only surprised; she found alpha lipoic's humble beginnings pretty funny, since I had her on a regimen that demanded that she give up one of her favorite foods — potatoes.

As I mentioned in a previous chapter, alpha lipoic acid is the universal antioxidant. It quickly penetrates the skin and enters all portions of a cell and begins to protect it from free-radical damage. In addition, alpha lipoic acid has the ability to increase energy production, helping the cells to repair themselves much more efficiently. Most important for Linda, however, was alpha lipoic's ability to reduce or eliminate inflammation. Her skin had developed a distinctly unattractive red, irritated look as a result of the irritating products she was slathering on it every other day. I promised her that the alpha lipoic acid would begin to improve the appearance of her skin in a matter of days.

I instructed her to wash with a mild, nondetergent cleanser twice a day. After each cleansing, she was to apply the alpha lipoic acid cream. If she still felt dry, she could use the fragrance-free moisturizer (since it's less irritating) of her choice. I also explained the importance of applying a sunscreen daily, once the alpha lipoic cream had been absorbed into her skin. Even though alpha lipoic acid is a powerful antioxidant that offers some protection from the free-radical damage of the sun, additional protection is needed.

Linda was then scheduled to return to my office in four weeks. By that time, I would have her lab test results as well as the details of the exam conducted by her internist.

Improving Linda's Body Chemistry

A few weeks later, a surprisingly upbeat Linda arrived at my office. Before she said a word, I could immediately see that her mood was far more positive. The first thing she said was, "I can already see a change in my skin, and I'm feeling much better." Her energy levels had increased, and, to her great surprise, she actually liked her new diet regimen. She had even devised her own system for taking her supplements so that she could stay on her vitamin program whether she was traveling or at home. She had come up with the idea of tucking each dose into little envelopes marked "a.m.," "lunch," or "p.m." to be sure she remained on schedule.

During the first part of her visit, I explained her lab test results. Linda had a slightly low red blood cell count (common among women who diet year-round), but she was not anemic. She also had a slightly low *BUN* level. The term *BUN* bears no relationship to the sticky delights of the same name: It is a measurement of *blood urea nitrogen*. Essentially, this reading tells us how much protein is being eliminated by the kidneys. If your BUN is very high, it means your kidneys are unable to remove protein from your body. Linda's blood also showed a low level of a protein called albumin. A decrease in serum albumin is associated with decreased life expectancy. The converse is also apparently true: People with high albumin levels are thought to live longer. Linda's level may have been on the low side because of her repeated history of infection and perhaps because of her extremely low protein diet.

The other lab result that grabbed my attention was Linda's DHEA level. It was extremely low. DHEA is a hormone produced by the adrenal gland. In our bodies, this hormone circulates at very high levels when we are young and tends to drop as we get older. Scientists have noticed a relationship between low DHEA levels and an increased risk of disease. This does not mean that low DHEA levels cause a number of diseases; it just means that there is an association. Many scientists suspect that people with higher DHEA levels are less likely to develop heart disease, arthritis, cancer, and many other conditions.

Since Linda had been under a great deal of stress, her body was producing large amounts of another hormone called *cortisol* — the stress response hormone. Whenever our bodies sense danger (read: "unwelcome stress") cortisol is secreted by the adrenal glands, which sit on top of the kidneys, to prepare us to do battle with an enemy. This is commonly referred to as the fight or flight response. The body's built-in defense system works wonders when you are seriously facing harm or injury, but problems arise when your cortisol levels remain high on a regular basis. That's what occurs when people are under chronic stress. When the body produces a constant cortisol overdose, muscle tissue begins to break down, blood sugar rises out of control, and even brain cells suffer damage.

We do not have all the answers about how

to prevent the adverse effects of stress, but we do know that DHEA helps the body fight the effects of high cortisol levels, which means it is an extremely important weapon to fight premature aging. Nothing can accelerate the aging process faster than stress, and cortisol is the key to that process.

For this reason, I suggested Linda begin supplementing her DHEA levels with a small daily dose. I would check her levels again in two months. One important point about DHEA: The supplement is best recommended by a physician, after your blood levels have been checked. I am very conservative about giving women DHEA, because it can be converted to testosterone and cause side effects such as excessive hair growth. Because DHEA is what we call a precursor hormone, it encourages the production of other hormones, and, therefore, it may increase levels of testosterone or estrogen, although the effect is different in everyone. I am very aware that DHEA is available in health food stores, but I do not recommend that consumers take high doses of the supplement under any circumstances. It's best to stick to a low dose (10 to 15 milligrams) and then only under the supervision of your health care professional.

The Final Pieces

Next, it was time to take a look at Linda's fitness program. Since she said she was feeling a little more energetic, I suggested she get back to her health club and begin a cross-training routine; that is, she would use a number of different types of exercise to strengthen her body in several ways. I suggested that she do weight-resistance exercises to build muscle strength, and cardiovascular exercises such as jogging, aerobics, or stairclimbing to bolster her heart, lungs, and stamina. I told her to begin slowly and not to increase the duration or intensity of her workouts by more than 10 percent in any one week.

Linda was happy to go along with my prescribed exercise regimen, so it was time to take an even closer look at her skin. After four weeks, the alpha lipoic acid had done an incredible job of reducing the inflammation. Linda's ruddy look was gone. In its place, she had a soft, radiant glow and a smoother complexion characterized by much smaller pores.

She was delighted with the results and very pleased to hear that the alpha lipoic acid had begun to repair her skin. In the coming months, her face would continue to look better.

She was also happy about the fact that her skin was firmer. I explained that the alpha lipoic acid cream also contained DMAE, which increases the tone of the skin (see Resources on page 262). After close examination, it was easy to see that Linda's jawline was more defined and her cheekbones were more prominent.

At this point, it was time to add topical vitamin C ester to her program. Unlike the vitamin C that she had been using when she first came to see me, this formula was not an acid and therefore would not irritate her skin. In addition, vitamin C ester can rapidly penetrate the skin because it is a fat-soluble rather than a water-soluble compound. Her collagen production would begin to increase, and that would add to the firmness and thickness of her skin.

Linda left my office with two important additions to her anti-aging program: a DHEA supplement and a vitamin C ester cream for nighttime use.

One Year Later, a Success

At the 12-month mark, Linda and I sat down to celebrate the many successes of her anti-aging program. First, her weight had remained steady at 135 pounds, but she was still ready to pick up a new wardrobe because she had lost so much body fat on her program. Her increased protein intake, exercise program, and improved nutrient profile had helped her to greatly increase her muscle mass, while getting rid of flab. Her energy level and performance at work had also improved dramatically.

But the most incredible difference was the change in her skin. The alpha lipoic acid/vitamin C ester combination had all but eliminated the fine lines from her 54-year-old complexion. And the discolorations brought on by her years of exposure to the sun were virtually invisible.

As effective as topical antioxidant creams and cleansers are, I must emphasize that part of Linda's new appearance was also attributable to the supplements she had been taking for cellular repair. Acetyl L-carnitine, for example, which was prescribed to help Linda with memory loss, is also known for its ability to reverse discoloration in the skin.

Her new round of lab tests also revealed that her DHEA and albumin levels were much closer to normal. And, thanks to her new diet, her red blood cell count had also increased.

Linda's results may seem unusual, but I commonly see similar responses in patients who stick with my anti-aging program. She was a prime example of anti-aging medicine at work.

Linda says she is now very proud that she has not only a much younger face, but a more youthful looking body as well. She happily credits her alpha lipoic acid body lotion, and vitamin C ester body cream (an added benefit of my program) for giving her softer, firmer, smoother skin from head to toe. Linda has actually witnessed the reversal of the aging process thanks to a total antioxidant program. And remember, her results are the norm, not the exception to the rule.

Anti-Aging Consultation 2: Harry

In many ways, Harry was a man doing an excellent job of managing the aging process. I first noticed him at my health club. At 69, Harry was known to give as good as he got on the racquetball court. I also discovered that he was an avid hiker who was as active as possible in just about every part of his life. But Harry's concerns about aging were quite different than Linda's. He was concerned about his appearance, but in addition to wanting to reduce the number of fine lines on his face and keep his skin firm, he was also fighting male pattern baldness and a pronounced loss of libido.

He came to me to address cosmetic concerns, but I assured him that with the cooperation of his internist, we could address his problems as a whole and help him keep the youthful lifestyle he wanted to maintain. Harry's only serious health problems were his elevated blood pressure and blood sugar. The medications prescribed by his internist were a problem, because they made him weak and tired. Harry dearly loved his active lifestyle, and he wanted to know if it was possible to deal with his health problems without having to endure the side effects of his medication.

Harry had one other concern. No matter how much he exercised, his weight was increasing. His internist had made it clear that the only way to keep his blood pressure and blood sugar under control was to keep his weight down. Since he was already very active and had such an optimistic, upbeat approach to life, Harry was interested in doing just about anything in his power to improve his health and maintain his vigorous lifestyle. Like Linda, he had even done his homework on anti-aging medicine (he'd attended a lecture or two) and was very interested in getting involved in a program.

Taking Stock

As always, the first step was to take a complete look at the patient's medical history and diet and exercise regimen. Harry made it easy for me. He immediately admitted that he just loved refined carbohydrates, like pasta. That would explain why he was 20 pounds overweight. A quick look at his background also revealed that his elevated blood sugar was owing to a combination of age, diet, and genetics.

I explained to Harry that as we age, our cells have a decreased ability to take in glucose, the form of sugar that circulates in our bloodstream. Therefore, we actually produce more insulin. Unfortunately, the insulin isn't as effective as it was in our youth at moving the sugar into our cells. That leaves us with blood that contains excess levels of glucose (sugar) and insulin. This combination is very detrimental to our blood vessels, heart, nerves, and kidneys. And even though we've come to think of sugar as a nutrient that increases energy, you actually have less energy when your body loses its ability to make use of the insulin in your blood. Abnormally high levels of blood sugar also set in motion another process that contributes to aging — free-radical production.

Harry's lab tests confirmed that he had high levels of blood sugar. They also showed that he had extremely low levels of testosterone and DHEA. Testosterone, the primary male sex hormone, declines with age just as the primary female sex hormone estrogen does. As the level of hormone drops, men experience a number of physical changes. Muscle and bone mass decrease, and that means that the skin starts to sag. The immune system weakens, and some men find it harder to concentrate or remember things. Testosterone is also responsible for balancing other hormones such as growth hormone, which can affect the amount of body fat that we burn. Low levels of the life-sustaining hormone are associated with a decreased resistance to disease.

Since Harry wanted to increase his athletic performance and counteract the negative effects of high blood sugar and high blood pressure, we launched a diet and supplements program targeted at these goals.

First, Harry was placed on a high-protein diet appropriate for his age, body weight, gender, and level of physical activity. I asked him to cut back on the refined carbohydrates (that meant saying good-bye to his beloved pasta) and eat more complex carbohydrates. The foods recommended for Harry were: salmon, swordfish, chicken, and turkey, as well as green salads, broccoli, cauliflower, squash, and limited amounts of lentils and beans.

His supplement program consisted of all of the most powerful antioxidants, including vitamins C and E, alpha lipoic acid, selenium, and CoQ_{10}. I prescribed CoQ_{10} at an extremely high level (300 milligrams daily) in order to counteract the effects of high blood sugar and high blood pressure. CoQ_{10} has been reported to help normalize blood pressure and assist in the regulation of blood sugar and protect the heart.

I also prescribed 300 milligrams of alpha lipoic acid a day, because alpha lipoic acid is extremely helpful for diabetics. Alpha lipoic acid, when taken orally, tends to counteract the negative effects of high blood sugar, while helping the body to get blood sugar levels under control. It can also reverse some of the nerve damage that is seen in patients with diabetes.

I then added an acetyl L-carnitine tablet to Harry's regimen to help protect his mitochondria from free-radical damage. Harry also took chromium, a trace mineral that can help normalize blood sugar. I then added DHEA, the mineral boron (which helps to promote testosterone production), as well as omega-3 fatty acids (fish oils) that would help his immune system and improve his ability to burn fat. I also placed him on calcium and magnesium supplements to keep his bones strong. And I told him to take a balance of B vitamins, including adequate amounts of B_6 and folic acid to help reduce his chances of developing heart disease.

And then we began testosterone supplements. I realize the use of testosterone supplements in men is somewhat controversial. However, testosterone is so important to maintaining normal body function — especially in an active male — that I feel it is essential to maintain normal levels. Harry's blood tests showed that his prostate was completely normal (testosterone can advance prostate cancer in high-risk individuals). Therefore, I started Harry on a testosterone gel cream, which he was to apply to his forearms once a day. This testosterone gel cream penetrates the skin and enters the bloodstream. The increase in testosterone level can be controlled merely by changing the amount of cream that is applied.

Finally, he was given supplements of conjugated linoleic acid (which help burn body fat and are helpful in weight reduction) and the amino acid taurine (which tends to be beneficial to the heart muscle; Harry's many activities suggested he required larger amounts of this amino acid).

As for dealing with Harry's skin, there are no surprises in what I recommended: a mix of the ingredients that we have talked about throughout this book, such as vitamin C ester and alpha lipoic acid containing DMAE applied topically.

Eighteen Months Later

Over the next 1½ years, I saw Harry on a monthly basis. Watching his progress was a wonderful experience. At an age when most people experience a steady decline in attractiveness and health, Harry was actually seeing his body improve each day. Thanks to applying topical alpha lipoic acid, as well as vitamin C ester, the lines and creases he had accumulated in years of outdoor sports had greatly softened. The skin on his face and jawline was also firmer than it had been in years. His blood pressure normalized, and he was eventually able to withdraw from his medications. The elevated levels of blood sugar improved greatly, and he found that he had more energy. Adding the testosterone and DHEA supplements also helped him to regain muscle mass.

At 71, Harry was in such good shape that his racquetball partners were complaining that he was winning too many games and making them look bad. After all, some of them are half his age!

Harry told me that he was quite pleased about the improvement in his sex life. His libido had increased, as well as his ability to perform. And one more thing. I do not claim that anti-aging medicine is a baldness cure, but Harry has noticed an extra tuft of hair or two since he began his program.

The last time I ran into Harry at the gym he had just returned from a mountain climbing expedition in Italy. He'd returned happy to report that he kept well ahead of the youngsters in the crowd. I was not surprised. The excess body fat that he had been lugging around at his first office visit had completely disappeared. Not only did Harry not feel 71; he looked like a man in his fifties.

Anti-Aging Consultation 3: Carter

There's nothing unusual about wanting to look your best. But for lots of baby boomers, the pressure to look young and vital comes from external sources, not internal motivation. For some, holding on to a hard-won career means staying quite a few steps (and often a few years) ahead of the competition. That was the situation facing Carter, who has been a patient of mine for more than seven years.

When I first began seeing him, Carter was a great-looking guy who had a few minor problems with eczema and an occasional plantar wart. He was a familiar face around Connecticut, where I have my practice, because he was a local television personality, a popular newscaster. Anyone who caught Carter on the evening news would have agreed that he was perfect for his job. He had thick, dark hair, steely blue eyes, a square jaw, and one of those deep, resonant voices that you only expect to hear emanating from a television or radio broadcast. As well-suited as he was for the job, the job was also perfectly suited for him. Carter loved his work.

One day, Carter walked into my office for an appointment. It had been about two years since his last visit, so I innocently asked what brought him in on this particular day. I was surprised at the answer. This visit certainly was not going to be about another outbreak of eczema. He started by saying he had been reading a lot about my anti-aging program in national magazines. He was subdued. His usual energy and optimism were absent. Something was definitely wrong.

After a few moments of polite conversation, Carter explained that his career was going downhill and he would no longer be featured regularly on the local television station. He had been shifted into a part-time reporting position.

No one at the station had been specific about the reasons for the change, but Carter thought it was related to his personal appearance — youthful appearance being an important requirement in television newscasters. Carter was only 44, but he was convinced that his face was aging. He knew that his body was no longer in the fit and trim condition it had been in just a few years ago. He was understandably upset and stressed out about his situation, and he wanted to know if I could help.

He was determined to get his career back on track, but he understood the television business well enough to know that he had to do something about his looks first.

Determining the Problem
It seemed that the job that Carter loved so much was also a primary contributor to his

looking older than his years. As I began to talk to him about diet and exercise, and as I set about updating his medical history, it was clear that he was not taking care of himself.

When he had first come to me as a patient, Carter had been extremely active. He ran nearly 25 miles per week. But as job pressures mounted, he could no longer find the time for exercise, so he just wasn't doing anything to keep fit. Since he was always dashing in and out of his office, or jumping on a plane, he had also begun eating most of his meals at fast-food restaurants — a habit he unfortunately kept up even when he was in between assignments. When he wasn't grabbing a burger, he was eating take-out from the canteen at work.

He was not taking any vitamin supplements, and he admitted that he would often work late or into the hours of the early morning and then return to work after getting just a couple of hours of sleep. One wouldn't need to be a health expert to see that stress, overwork, and poor eating and exercise habits were putting Carter on the fast track to premature aging.

I explained to Carter that I wanted to get some basic laboratory tests run and have him return in a week. At that point we could discuss the findings as well as outline a program to help him get his life back.

The laboratory studies were unremarkable, with results indicating a basically healthy man. But Carter's cortisol levels were well above normal, which meant that he was under a great deal of stress. Chronically elevated cortisol is extremely harmful to us on many levels. As mentioned in the case study of Linda a few pages back, when your cortisol goes up, your brain cells are at increased risk for damage, and your blood sugar rises as well. Your chances of developing high blood pressure and heart disease increase, and you become much more susceptible to infections. Working to bring Carter's cortisol levels down into a healthy range was going to be a critical part of his anti-aging program.

The First Steps

When I asked Carter to tell me his chief concerns — other than wanting his career back, of course — he said he wanted to do something about looking so much older. After a close physical examination, I had to agree with him. His complexion, which had once been healthy and clear, looked sallow and dull. Fine lines were beginning to creep in around his eyes, and he was developing furrows in his forehead. His once crisp jawline was also beginning to sag in a few places, so his face looked aged in person and on camera. And his once-trim runner's physique was slowly being replaced by a flabby body, characterized by a spreading midsection.

After conducting a physical exam, I explained to Carter that before he did anything, he absolutely had to drop his junk-food diet. I went on to tell him that not only would a diet high in nutrients and low in fat begin to take the extra inches off his stomach; it would also have a calming, anti-inflammatory effect on his body, slowing the overall process of aging.

Carter was skeptical that diet could achieve this magical goal, but he was more than willing to listen. Once we got him off his nearly daily doses of high-fat, take-out fare, I intended to put him on a nutritional supplement program that would improve his skin, help him drop some weight, as well as help him think faster and more clearly.

The first thing I asked him to do was surprisingly simple. After talking with him, it became clear that he seldom drank enough water. So for his first major step toward a younger body, mind, and spirit, I asked him to drink eight to ten glasses of water per day.

Carter was shocked to hear that water could make a difference in his health, but he agreed to go along. Of course, water is more than just something to quench your thirst. It's the universal solvent, carrying nutrients to every cell in our body, flushing out the toxins, and improving the functioning of our immune system. Good hydration also helps your skin and other organs stay healthy. Believe it or not, most people walk around in a state of mild dehydration at all times.

Eating for Longevity

Carter's diet makeover began with a recommendation that he eat a healthy breakfast each day that would boost his energy and help him resist his junk-food cravings. The most important part of his morning meal would be protein — high-quality protein that is low in fat (indeed, most animal fats are pro-inflammatory and tend to accelerate aging). I like protein in the morning — such as salmon or scrambled egg whites — because it doesn't increase blood sugar levels.

Next, I explained to Carter the importance of keeping his insulin levels in check by decreasing his intake of refined carbohydrates and increasing his protein intake.

Like most of my patients, Carter was unaware that high levels of insulin in the body can be extremely harmful — even in people who are not diabetic. We know that insulin, secreted in response to eating refined carbohydrates or sugars, can lead to inflammation within every cell of the body. In addition, insulin causes fat to be stored in the lining of our arteries, which can lead to high blood pressure and clogging of the arteries to the heart.

Last, I made it clear that carbohydrates make it possible for us to have the energy we need to get through the day and maintain stable blood sugar — but we have to eat the *right* carbohydrates.

A drop in blood sugar can do more than leave you sleepy in the afternoon. It can leave your complexion looking drawn and dull. And that's the last thing you need if you're standing in front of a television camera every day. So to get Carter's day off to a high-energy start and keep him feeling balanced throughout the day, I suggested that he try eating a complex carbohydrate, such as a bowl of oatmeal, or fresh blueberries or strawberries, each morning with his protein component.

Finally, I mentioned that it is important to have some fat in the diet. Carter was confused, since I had already told him that fats were pro-inflammatory. But like most people, he didn't know the difference between good fats and bad fats. I talked about this earlier in the book, but there's one more bit of knowledge you need to have in order to understand about the "good fat" — essential fatty acids (EFAs): There are two types: omega-3 and omega-6. We all need a balance of omega-6 and omega-3 fatty acids in our bodies to stay well. But the average American diet consists of very high levels of omega-6 alone, which can often lead to a pro-inflammatory state.

Omega-3, the fatty acid many of us need more of, is found in high levels in fish. That's why I suggested to Carter that he add a little nontraditional food, such as grilled salmon, to his breakfast menu. Salmon, in addition to being a high-quality protein, also has high levels of omega-3 oils, as do many of the cold water fish. In addition, fish contains high levels of a substance call DMAE that enhances cognitive function, as we learned a few pages ago.

Carter was a bit overwhelmed by the idea of sorting types of fat every time he sat down to a meal, so I asked him to try to remember these simple guidelines: Bad fat is generally fat that's solid at room temperature — margarines, butter, and animal fats — as well as anything that says "hydrogenated" on the package. Good fats are a part of healthy foods, such as fish, low-fat meats such as turkey and white-meat chicken, and oils like olive oil. To be absolutely sure that he was getting the right amount of essential fatty acids, I added supplements to his diet, such as flaxseed oil (which contains a lot of alpha-linolenic acid) and borage oil (which contain high amounts of gamma-linolenic acid).

When we were through, Carter was armed with more than a complete education about nutrition. He also understood why the fast food he had been grabbing day after day was not just making him fat; it was draining his energy and adding years to his looks. That knowledge was the extra incentive he needed to dedicate himself to a high-protein, moderate-carbohydrate regimen that was far lower in saturated fats and sugars than his old diet had been. Once his eating was under control, it was time to address his weight and skin problems.

Slimming That Spare Tire

As a former runner, Carter was already sold on the importance of exercise. His only problem was finding the energy and discipline to get back to a healthy routine. He knew he would look and feel much better if he returned to running three to four miles, five times a week. To give him a little extra encouragement, I talked with him briefly about how exercise increases circulation, helps us to utilize nutrients better, and keeps blood sugar levels in balance.

And if that didn't get him into his running shoes and back out on the track, I reminded him that there are piles of reputable studies showing that the onset of virtually every chronic disease can be delayed or avoided through regular exercise. Exercise is a critical part of any anti-aging program, and for Carter it would be the quickest way to bring a healthier glow back to his skin and to lower his body fat.

I suggested that in addition to his running, he add a weight-lifting program to increase muscle mass. We now know that the larger amount of muscle mass we have, the better our ability to utilize calories and the greater our resistance to diabetes and other illnesses. Weight-bearing exercise also keeps our bones healthy and helps prevent injury and fractures.

In addition to a regular exercise program and a good diet, I felt that at age 44 Carter would benefit greatly from a very aggressive nutritional supplement program. Carter was very aware of the connection between free radicals and the aging process, and he was also aware of the benefits of antioxidants, since he had just completed an investigative news story on the subject. As with my other patients, the supplements program I prescribed was detailed, but for good reason. The list below starts with the antioxidants I suggested for Carter, followed by other vitamins, minerals, natural supplements, and one herbal extract — all of which have beneficial effects that were well suited to Carter's goals.

- Vitamin C, 1,000 milligrams, three times a day. I told Carter to take each pill 30 minutes before eating. As you know, vitamin C is excellent for building the immune system and preventing free-radical damage. There also is some fairly good evidence that taking oral vitamin C can help decrease the incidence of skin cancer.
- Coenzyme Q_{10}, 30 milligrams, twice daily. CoQ_{10} is an excellent antioxidant that also helps to protect the heart.
- Alpha lipoic acid supplement, 100 milligrams a day. This supplement would help Carter fight all of the inflammatory

processes that come with stress and aging.

- Selenium, 200 micrograms daily. I added this supplement because it too is a good antioxidant.
- Vitamin E-gamma and mixed tocopherol type, 400 milligrams daily
- Vitamin E-tocotrienol type, 100 milligrams daily
- DMAE, 100 milligrams daily. In addition to the DMAE that Carter would be obtaining in his diet, I asked him to take a supplement as well in order to increase his mental abilities and help him with work.
- Conjugated linoleic acid, 2,000 milligrams daily. Conjugated linoleic acids help us to lose body fat rapidly and prevent some bowel cancers.
- Acetyl L-carnitine, 1,000 milligrams daily. I recommended this supplement to help Carter improve his physical performance and burn off flab. Research also shows that L-carnitine rapidly penetrates the blood-brain barrier and does a wonderful job of improving cognitive function.
- Chromium picolinate, 200 micrograms daily. This supplement would help stabilize Carter's blood sugar levels.

- Vitamin B_5 (also known as pantothenic acid), 500 milligrams daily. I recommended this B vitamin to counteract some of the effects of the stress he was under and to lower his elevated cortisol levels.
- A balanced B-vitamin supplement containing fairly high amounts of the B-complex vitamins, such as B_1 (50 milligrams), B_2 (25 milligrams), B_3 (25 milligrams), B_6 (25 milligrams), folic acid (800 micrograms), and B_{12} (500 micrograms).
- Magnesium aspartate, 300 milligrams daily
- Magnesium succinate, 300 milligrams daily
- Potassium aspartate, 150 milligrams, daily

The last three minerals were added because they help us metabolize calories and also make the heart healthier.

- Calcium carbonate, 1,000 milligrams daily. I strongly believe in supplementing calcium in both men and women to prevent future osteoporosis.
- Ginkgo biloba, 60 milligrams a day, to be taken in the morning. This herbal

supplement improves cognitive enhancement.

Creating a Camera-Ready Complexion

Once I was sure that I had created a solid nutritional foundation for Carter's anti-aging program and convinced him of the importance of returning to his workout regimen, I could be sure that he would get the best possible results from his topical skin care plan.

He had two unique problems that needed to be resolved in addition to the basic aging issues we all face. First, he needed a quick response from his skin care products. His career was on hold, and he needed to get back in gear. Second, he had to look good under hot television lights, and maintain a healthy complexion even though he was slathering on heavy stage makeup whenever he went on the air. This made putting together a workable plan for him a challenge, but I was sure the proper antioxidant combinations would do the trick.

First, I asked him to get into the habit of washing his face with a special nonirritating cleanser that would help prevent inflammation and remove all traces of pancake makeup from his skin after broadcasts. I then showed him how to produce the face-lift effect that several of my clients who have on-camera careers swear by — a combination of vitamin C ester cream containing a high-potency DMAE complex cream. This powerful antioxidant duo creates the almost immediate face-lift effect that I explained in chapter 7 — an instant youth boost that would greatly enhance Carter's appearance on the air.

Carter thought that I had to be kidding. He just did not believe that any skin care product could make that kind of a difference. So he sat there patiently as I poured a small amount of DMAE/vitamin C ester mix into my hand and applied it to the left side of his face, beginning at the hairline. I smoothed the cream down his cheek, underneath his chin, onto his neck, and up behind his ears, making sure I covered only half of his face. In order for him to see the full effect, I left the right side of his face untreated. We then sat and talked about his daily regimen.

While we waited for results, I told Carter that he should get into the habit of applying the DMAE/vitamin C ester formula at least 30 minutes before appearing on camera. This would give the formula's active ingredients enough time to improve his skin tone, giving him a firmer chin line and a fresher, younger look on the air. In addition, I suggested that Carter begin using alpha lipoic acid on his face and neck twice daily. Alpha lipoic acid would help diminish lines and wrinkles and some of the imperfections that Carter was beginning to see each day. It would also reduce some of the puffiness that he was noticing underneath his eyes, as well as help lighten the dark circles he was starting to develop. Alpha lipoic acid also tends to make the pores tighter and give the skin a porcelain-like appearance.

I advised him to apply the alpha lipoic acid cream mornings and evenings, after mild cleansings. He should begin with an application every other day, so that his skin could become accustomed to the lotion. If he experienced no irritation after the first week, then he could apply the cream every day for the second week. Finally, if no irritation developed after the second week, he would then move up to a twice-a-day regimen. By going slowly with this very powerful product, he would get maximum benefits without showing any signs of irritation.

About 25 minutes had passed since I had applied the DMAE/vitamin C ester formula, so I handed Carter a mirror and asked him to look at the results. The look on his face said it all. He was amazed at the difference between the right and left sides. On the left side of his face, his eye was wide open and the lid had a much tighter appearance than the lid on the right side. His nasolabial fold (that line that etches itself into the face in the space between the base of the nose and the corners of the mouth, adding years to your appearance) was greatly diminished, and his jawline was sharper. I was very pleased to see that even his left cheekbone was a bit more prominent than the right.

Carter also noticed that his neck looked much smoother despite all the sun damage he had sustained over the years. Carter stared at the mirror for several minutes and looked at me and asked, "Where has this science been all my life?"

After making sure that I applied the DMAE/vitamin C ester complex to the other side of his face, we scheduled a follow-up visit so that I could check on his progress.

Regaining His Stride

Upon his follow-up visit, Carter was more relaxed looking than I had ever seen him. His old enthusiasm, smile, and optimism had also returned. As we sat down to talk, he just couldn't wait to tell me about how his life had changed in the past 30 days.

First of all, he said that he had left my office and gone directly to the vitamin store to get his supplement program started. Within a day or two, he went back to his local health club to begin a weight-lifting program to complement his new jogging routine. He couldn't say enough about his increased energy level, and he was sleeping much better as well.

A decline in fat and an increase in muscle tissue were beginning to take inches off his waist. He was also pleased and surprised to discover that his workout recovery time was half of what it had been even when he was a much younger man. I explained that this was his nutrition and supplement program at work, helping his body get back into shape.

The best and most important news, however, was about his career. He could see from his tapes that he was looking a lot better on camera (he always uses his DMAE/vitamin C ester cream before stepping in front of the lights). His makeup person and his producer had even commented on how good he looked. His really big news, however, was that he was feeling confident enough to go for a job interview in the area's top news market — New York

City. He had a shot at a possible position as a regular on a network show.

A few weeks later, I got the call. Carter got the job in New York. He had successfully recovered his career. Now, whenever he's in town he stops by to say hello and show off the results of his continued dedication to his anti-aging program. He actually looks years younger than he did that day when he came in for his first anti-aging consultation. And he's become so passionate about his fitness routine that he finished the New York City Marathon in a very respectable time, and sincerely plans on running every year until his eighties.

Carter also started another behind-the-scenes trend. When his fellow newscasters found out about the DMAE/vitamin C ester formula, word spread from TV station to TV station with the speed of a breaking story. Now, anchors all over the country consider DMAE/vitamin C ester formula a critical part of their routine for looking their best on the air.

Happy Endings

As you can see, Linda, Harry, and Carter had very different issues related to health and their appearance, but the science of anti-aging medicine helped all three of them address and relieve many of the concerns that people think are just hopeless at their stage of life.

What's all of this got to do with having beautiful, wrinkle-free skin? Everything. You see, protecting your youthful appearance is a holistic process. I could have given Linda and Harry an armload of creams and cleansers and sent them on their way, but then I would have addressed only half of their concerns. I've made this point throughout this book, but it's so important that it needs to be repeated: To keep your skin gorgeous, young, and smooth on the outside, you must work on the inside of your body as well. That's why I strongly recommend that you begin your *Wrinkle Cure* program with a full, anti-aging medical consultation so that you can fully benefit from recent antioxidant discoveries and look and feel your best well into your later years.

Chapter 12

Facing

the Future

Spin Traps: Stopping Free-Radical Damage Before It Begins

A single image could easily dominate the concept of antioxidants at work against free radicals: a team of assorted emergency workers scurrying across a disaster-torn cellular landscape, rushing from place to place to heal the wounded, shore up crumbling structures, and stop the next disaster before it strikes again.

Until now, free radicals have basically been in control in the battle against aging. Yes, antioxidants have given us a method for slowing or mending free-radical damage, but we have yet to master a method for rendering this destructive molecule powerless. That is until now.

Thanks to a peculiar-sounding chemical substance called a spin trap, we will make quantum leaps in the effort to control the effects of aging in the new millennium. *Spin traps* are chemicals that create a barrier — a trap — that holds free radicals in place so that they can be studied, tracked, and stopped, before they scar the cells that make up your skin. Here's how they work.

A New Kind of Protection

In order to be able to really understand the type and scope of damage that free radicals can cause in a cell, scientists decided that they needed a method for observing and measuring free-radical activity in a living system.

They solved the problem by using chemicals that could trap free radicals so that they could be measured using various instruments — in this case, chemicals whose molecules would join with free radicals, and then send off a sort of magnetic signal that could then be measured using a system called electron paramagnetic resonance. Since the measurement process is called electron spin resonance, the name *spin trap* was born. This research was originally intended to help physicians and scientists detect the presence of free radicals when certain health problems were present in the human body. As they worked, however, the researchers found that the traps actually prevented the free radicals from moving from place to place and damaging cells. The substances used as spin traps were not particularly exotic, but it was quickly understood that they had enormous potential for helping us stay healthy.

One of the most frequently used spin traps is a substance called phenylbutyl nitrone (PBN). This chemical was initially tested in animals to see if it could reverse aging in the brain. Two scientists — Pamela E. Starke-Reed, Ph.D., director of nutrition at the National Institute on Aging, and John Carney, Ph.D., chief technical officer at Centaur Pharmaceuticals, who collaborates with researchers at the University of Kentucky in Lexington — gave a PBN dietary supplement to gerbils and then tested their intelligence after a two-week period by timing the gerbils' trips through a maze. Prior to the PBN diet regimen, the younger animals consistently completed the maze much faster than the older animals. When the older animals were tested after receiving PBN, they ran the maze as efficiently as the young animals. The scientists concluded that a reversal of brain aging had taken place, due to the antioxidant effects of PBN.

Currently, PBN and other chemical derivatives of the nitrone class are being tested in humans to treat stroke. When a person suffers from a stroke, the brain is briefly deprived of oxygen, because of circulatory problems. When the blood flow normalizes, oxygen is again present, and a great number of free-radical species are produced. These free radicals then do damage to the delicate brain tissue. When scientists administered nitrone spin traps to patients with stroke, the incidence of paralysis and speech problems was much decreased owing to the protective effect of this amazing chemical. Carney explained that it was protection against the oxidative damage to the central nervous system by PBN and other spin-trapping agents that accounts for the chemical's efficacy in treating the effects of stroke.

Phenylbutyl nitrone was one of the first spin traps tested and used in animals. Since these early studies in 1990, other nitrones have been synthesized and isolated that show activity 10 to 20 times greater than PBN. We have only just begun to investigate the power of nitrone spin traps to rejuvenate and protect the skin, but preliminary study results have been impressive. Nitrone spin traps show great anti-inflammatory activity on skin and, as you certainly know by now, inflammation equals aging. It is logical to assume that the anti-inflammatory activity of the nitrones would be owing to their ability to neutralize free radicals in the skin.

Scientists anticipate that someday nitrones will bring about dramatic improvements in the appearance of the lines, wrinkles, and sagging jowls found in older skin. So although spin traps may sound like some clever maneuver best suited to a video game, the odds are these free-radical fighters will become a highly effective method of maintaining a youthful, radiant complexion throughout life.

Telomerase: Staying Forever Young

In chapter after chapter, I've worked hard to emphasize that hard science is behind every highly effective skin care product — no smoke, no mirrors, no magic.

It may seem strange, then, at the close of this book, to call to mind a concept as romantic and steeped in fantasy as eternal youth. In many ways, however, that is exactly where anti-aging research is taking us. In just ten years, we may be able to permanently erase wrinkles from our skin, or stop them before they start, with nothing more than a well-formulated lotion or cream. Someday we may know how to delay, or postpone indefinitely, the sagging jaws, sallow complexions, age spots, and graying hair we've come to expect after the fourth or fifth decade of life. The technology and the knowledge is within our grasp.

The latest discovery of how to prolong life comes from a very surprising source. Very early in *The Wrinkle Cure* I explained that all cells have a finite lifespan. The single exception to this rule is cancer cells, which are immortal, despite the fact that they so often bring an end to life. A group of scientists has discovered how to nurture and protect life with the help of these immortal cells. Their research is focused on a single enzyme called *telomerase*.

Researchers have known for years that cells cannot divide indefinitely. Previously, I discussed the fact that after a certain number of divisions, cells become senescent — and stop dividing. One of the theories of aging is that senescence occurs because of the loss of a portion of the chromosome called *telomeres*. Each time a cell divides, it loses a tiny portion of a sort of tail called the *telomere*. Once the telomere shortens to a certain point, the cell loses its ability to divide, and it becomes senescent. The rate at which the telomere degrades is even used as a timing device to determine the lifespan of a cell.

Cancer cells are unique because they contain the enzyme telomerase, which can add DNA to the telomeres, lengthening them and allowing cells to divide indefinitely.

Researchers have suspected that if they could find a way to introduce telomerase into healthy cells, they could prolong the lifespan of the normal cells in the body. A recent study, reported in the *Journal of Science* by Jerry Shay, Ph.D., a professor at the University of Texas Southwestern Medical Center, found that a new genetic engineering technology makes it possible to introduce the enzyme telomerase into normal human dermal fibroblasts — the cells that make collagen and elastin in our skin.

Once Shay gave these fibroblasts the ability to produce telomerase, he placed them in cell cultures in a test tube. He then counted the number of cell divisions while comparing them to fibroblasts being maintained in identical cell cultures that did not have the ability to produce telomerase. The telomerase-producing fibroblasts achieved more than double the number of divisions compared to the untreated cells — an accomplishment that led Shay, and other scientists, to declare the treated cells immortal.

The research caused such excitement in

the medical community that a company called the Geron Corporation decided to work with the doctors at Southwestern Medical Center in an effort to produce a telomerase-based anti-aging therapy.

The one pressing question on every scientist's mind as this research progresses is: "Can the introduction of telomerase into a normal cell result in cancer, since cancer cells express this enzyme?" So far, the results of the cell culture studies using the skin fibroblasts show no abnormalities, and scientists are optimistic that using telomerase to produce perpetually healthy cells is safe. There is also work under way to investigate ways of removing telomerase from cancer cells in an effort to stop the disease.

When can you expect to be able to request telomerase-based anti-aging therapy from your doctor? Most scientists believe that in just 5 to 10 years, we will all be able to benefit from this discovery. But we already have the ability to introduce telomerase into skin cells using a topical lotion that contains liposomes, tiny capsules that can penetrate the cell membrane.

Although more research needs to be done to prove the effectiveness of this approach, if the body's skin cells respond to the telomerase in the same way as the cells treated by Shay, the result would be permanently youthful skin.

Telomerase just may be the basis for the ultimate anti-aging cream. Even telomerase, however, could not perform this miracle alone. Aging is a multifaceted phenomenon, so it would still be important to battle free radicals to keep your skin beautiful and your body disease-free. Combining telomerase, then, with the antioxidants discovered in just the past few years might eliminate altogether the damage that comes with age.

It is ironic that studying cancer could lead to a major breakthrough in lengthening the life of healthy cells. The study of aging, however, is filled with paradoxes and surprises. Oxygen, which is essential to support life, is also the major source of free radicals, which are partially responsible for many degenerative diseases. The greater the energy production in the cell, the more free radicals are produced, yet aging cells are characterized by decreased energy production — and the list goes on.

As you can see, the antioxidant revolution is just the beginning. Today's tocotrienol, spin trap, and telomerase discoveries are giant steps toward solving tomorrow's big questions about how and why we grow old.

Thanks to the antioxidant revolution, you now possess nature's secrets to keeping your skin smooth, supple, glowing, and virtually line-free for decades to come, while you protect your health and vitality with your own, personal, anti-aging plan. I know that the vitamins and other nutrients I've introduced you to in these pages will greatly improve the appearance of your skin, no matter how old you are. How can I be so sure? I've seen miraculous changes in my patients' complexions, and often their lives, as a result of topical and oral antioxidant-based treatment regimes. So much so, in fact, that I am continuing my research into the powers of vitamin C, vitamin E, alpha lipoic acid, and alpha hydroxy acids, while constantly searching for even better solutions to the problems of aging skin. I'm convinced that the antioxidant revolution is just beginning. Each triumph brings us one step closer to making the fantasy of eternal youth and beauty a realistic and obtainable goal.

Resources

Vitamin C Ester Products
- Selected Nordstrom Stores
- Nordstrom Beauty Hotline: (800) 7BEAUTY
- www.nvperriconemd.com
- Clinical Creations, LLC: (888) 823-7837
- Sephora Stores
- www.Sephora.com
- Selected Saks 5th Avenue Stores
- Jan Marini Skin Research, Inc.: through doctors' offices only

Alpha Lipoic Acid Products
- Selected Nordstrom Stores
- Nordstrom Beauty Hotline: (800) 7BEAUTY
- www.nvperriconemd.com
- Clinical Creations, LLC: (888) 823-7837
- Sephora Stores
- www.Sephora.com
- Selected Saks 5th Avenue Stores
- Selected plastic surgeons' offices

DMAE Products (NTP Complex)
- Selected Nordstrom Stores
- Nordstrom Beauty Hotline: (800) 7BEAUTY
- www.nvperriconemd.com
- Clinical Creations, LLC: (888) 823-7837
- Sephora Stores
- www.Sephora.com
- Selected Saks 5th Avenue Stores

Alpha Hydroxy Acid Products
- Aqua Glycolic brand: available in pharmacies
- Pond's Age Defying Complex: available in pharmacies
- At Home Products
- Avon Anew All-In-One Intensive Complex
- Physicians' offices
  Jan Marini Skin Research Products: (800) 347-2223
- Glyderm: (800) 321-4576
  M.D. Forte — (800) 253-9499
  Murad (physicians/aestheticians): (800) 33MURAD

Vitamin Supplements
- Bronson Pharmaceuticals
  A complete line of high-quality vita-

mins and minerals at excellent prices
- Optimum Health: (800) 228-1507

  Vitamin tablets that contain balanced formulas of essential nutrients and antioxidants

  Excellent source for Coenzyme Q_{10} that is highly bioavailable

  Liquid Calcium

  Flora Therapy

  Carni Q-Gel+

  Q-Gel Power

  Physicians Super Antioxidant Vitamin, Mineral & Phyto-Nutrient Active Formula
- NVPerricone Nutriceuticals

  Skin Foods drinks containing optimum levels of vitamins, minerals, protein, and carbohydrates for beautiful skin and a healthy body, www.nvperriconemd.com

Coenzyme Q_{10} Cream
- Beiersdorf
- Nivea Visage Wrinkle Control Q_{10}
- Juvena www.sephora.com
-

Cleansers
- Cetaphil, liquid and bar
- Dove Beauty Bar
- Oil of Olay Beauty Bar

- Basis Sensitive Skin Bar
- Neutrogena Non-Drying Cleansing Lotion

Moisturizers for Oily Skin
- Alpha Hydrox Oil-Free Lotion
- Prescriptives All You Need For Oily Skin

Moisturizers for Normal to Dry Skin
- Neutrogena Healthy Skin Face Lotion
- Oil of Olay Daily UV Protectant Beauty Fluid
- Pen Kera Lotion
- Eucerin Face Cream

Sunscreens
Minimum recommendation is SPF-15. An abbreviated list of companies offering excellent sunscreens:
- Westwood-Squibb PreSun products
- Hawaiian Tropic Sunscreen products
- Sun Pharmaceuticals/Banana Boat products
- Schering Plough/Coppertone products
- Proctor & Gamble/Oil of Olay UV Protectant
- Estee Lauder Advanced Sun Care products
- Fisher Pharmaceuticals/Ti Screen

- Beiersdorf/Eucerin Daily Facial Lotion
- Avon Products/Anew and Sunseekers

Copper Peptide Complex Skin Cream
- Skin Biology, Inc.: (800) 405-1912
- Protect & Restore Skin Renewal Cream

Anti-Aging Doctors
- American Academy of Anti-Aging Medicine: (773) 528-4333 or www.worldhealth.net
- Directory of Innovative Doctors
    Published by the Life Extension Foundation: (800) 544-4440 or www.lef.org (click on "Innovative Doctors")

References

Chapter 2

Textbook of Dermatology, edited by Arthur Rook, D. S. Wilkinson and S. J. G. Ebling. Volume 1, 3rd edition. "The Normal Skin," pages 5–30. 1968.

A. K. Balan, A. M. Kligman. *Skin and Aging*. New York: Raven Press, 1989.

The Biologic Effects of Ultraviolet Radiation, edited by F. Urbach. Oxford Pergamon Press. 1969.

G. J. Fisher, Z. Q. Wang, S. C. Daha, S. Kang, J. J. Voorhees. "Pathophysiology of Premature Skin Aging Induced By Ultraviolet Light." *New England Journal of Medicine.* 1997; 337: 1419–1429.

Chapter 3

Kligman, L. H. "Skin Changes in Photoaging: Characteristics, Prevention and Repair." In *Skin and Aging*. A. K. Balan and A. M. Kligman, editors. New York: Raven Press, 1989: 331–346.

Chapter 4

Nagy, I. *The Membrane Hypothesis of Aging*. CRC Press. 1994.

Hayflick, L. "The Limited In Vitro Lifetime of Human Diploid Cell Strains," *Exp. Cell Res.*, 37, 614–636.

Harman, D. "Free Radical Theory of Aging: Current Status," In *Lipofuscin — 1987: State of the Art, 1*.

Pathak, M. A.; Stratton, K. "Effects of Ultraviolet and Visible Radiation and the Production of Free Radicals in Skin." In *Biologic Effects of Ultraviolet Radiation*, F. Urbach, editor. Oxford Pergamon Press, 1969: 207.

Chapter 5

Fann, Y. D.; Rothbert, K. B.; Tremml, J. S.; Douglas, A.; DuBois, B. "Ascorbic Acid Promotes Prostanoid Release in Human Lung Parenchyma." *Prostaglandins*. 1986; 31: 361–368.

Ogilvy, C. S.; DuBois, A.; Douglas, J. "Effects of Ascorbic Acid and Endomethicin on the Airway of Healthy Male Subjects With and Without Induced Bronchial Constriction." *J. Allergy Clin. Immunol.* 1981; 67: 363–369.

Perricone, N. V. "Treatment of Psoriasis With Topical Ascorbyl Palmitate." *Clinical Research*. 1991; 39:535A Abstract.

Perricone, N. V. "Photoprotective and Anti-Inflammatory Effects of Topical Ascorbyl Palmitate." *J. Ger. Derm.* 1993; 1 (1:5–10).

Vitamin C in Health and Disease, edited by Lester Packer and Jürgen Fuchs. New York: Marcel Dekker, 1997.

Smart, R.; Crawford, C. L. "Effect of Ascorbic Acid in its Synthetic Lipophilic Derivative Ascorbyl Palmitate in Phorbol Ester Induced Skin Tumor Promotion In Mice." *Am. J. Clin. Nutr.* 1991; 54: 1266S.

Chapter 6

Lipoic Acid in Health and Disease, edited by Jürgen Fuchs, Lester Packer and Guido Zimmer. New York: Marcel Dekker, 1997.

Fuchs J.; Milbradt, R. "Antioxidant Inhibition of Skin Inflammation Induced By Reactive Oxidants: Evaluation of the Redox Couple Dihydrolipoate/Lipoate." *Skin Pharmacol.* 1994; 7:278–284.

Podda, M.; Rallis, M.; Traber, M. G.; et al. "Kinetic Study of Cutaneous and Subcutaneous Distribution Following Topical Application of (7,8–14C) RAC–Alpha Lipoic Acid Onto Hairless Mice." *Biochem. Pharmacol.* 1996; 52: 627–633.

Chapter 7

Perricone, N. V. "Topical Vitamin C Ester (Ascorbyl Palmitate)" adapted from The First Annual Symposium on Aging Skin, San Diego, CA. *J. Ger. Dermatol.*

1997; 5(4):162–170.

Stryer, L. *Biochemistry, 3rd edition*. San Francisco: Freeman, 1988.

Murase, K.; Hattori, A.; Kohno, M.; Hayashi, K. "Stimulation of Nerve Growth Factor Synthesis/Secretion in Mouse Astroglial Cells By Co-Enzymes." *Biochem. Mol. Biol. Int.* 1993; 30: 615–621.

Spencer, P. S.; Sabri, M. I.; Schaumburg, H. H. "Does A Defect of Energy Metabolism In the Nerve Fiber Underlie Axonal Degeneration And Polyneuropathies?" *Ann. Neurol.* 1979; 5: 501–507.

Guyton, Arthur C., *Textbook of Medical Physiology*, Chapter 11 "Contraction of Skeletal Muscle." pp. 131–147. Philadelphia: W.B. Saunders Co., 1971.

Chapter 8

Perricone, N. V.; DiNardo, J. C. "The Photoprotective and Anti-Inflammatory Effects of Topical Glycolic Acid." *Derm. Surgery*, Vol. 22, No. 5, May 1996. 435–437.

Van Scott, E. J.; Yu, R. J. "Hyperkeratinization, Corneocyte Cohesion and Alpha Hydroxy Acids." *J. Am. Acad. Dermatol.* 1984; 11: 867–79.

Sinatra, Steven T. *The Coenzyme Q_{10} Phenomenon*. Chicago: Keats Publishing, 1998.

Goodman, L. S. and Gilman, A., *The*

Pharmacologic Basis of Therapeutics, 5th edition. New York: Macmillan Publishing Company, 1975.

Chapter 9

Bodnar, Andrea G.; Ouellette, Michel; Frolkis, Maria; Holt, Shawn E.; Chiu, Choy-Pik; Morin, Gregg B.; Harley, Calvin B.; Shay, Jerry W.; Lichtsteiner, Serge; Wright, Woodring E. "Extension of Life-Span by Introduction of Telomerase into Normal Human Cells." *Science.* 16 January 1998, 279:349–52.

Chapter 10

Block, G. "The Data Support a Role for Antioxidants in Reducing Cancer Risk." *Nutr. Rev.* 50:207–213 (1992).

Jacob, R. A. et al. "Immunocompetence and Oxidant Defense During Ascorbate Depletion of Healthy Men." *Am. J. Clin. Nutr.* 54:1302S–1309S (1991).

Meadows, G. G. et al. "Ascorbate in the Treatment of Experimental Transplanted Melanoma." *Am. J. Clin. Nutr.* 54:1284S–91S (1991).

Perricone, N. V. "The Photoprotective and Anti-Inflammatory Effects of Topical Ascorbyl Palmitate." *J. Ger. Derm.* 1:1, 5–10 (Spring, 1993).

Burton, G. W., et al. "Autoxidation of Biological Molecules 4: Maximizing the Antioxidant Activity of Phenols." *J. Am. Chem. Soc.* 107: 7053–7065 (1985).

The Merck Index, 11th ed., entries 9417–9423 and 9931 (1989).

Nakano, M., et al. "Interaction Between an Organic Hydroperoxide and an Unsaturated Phospholipid and Alpha-Tocopherol in Model Membranes." *Biochim Biophys. Acta* 619: 274–286 (1980).

Serbinova, E., et al. "Free Radical Recycling and Intermembrane Mobility in the Antioxidant Properties of Alpha Tocopherol and Alpha-Tocotrienol." *Free Radical Biology & Med.* 10:263–275 (1991).

Wilson, R. "Antioxidants to Augment the Efficacy of Sunscreens." *Drug and Cosmetic Industry* 151:32-34, 38 and 68 (Aug. 1992).

Chapter 11

Sinatra, Steven, *Optimum Health*. New York: Bantam Books, 1998.

Passwater, Richard A., *The New Supernutrition*. New York: Pocket Books, 1991.

Chapter 12

Carney and Floyd, "Protection Against Oxidative Damage to CNS by PBN and Other Spin-Trapping Agents: A Novel

Series of Nonlipid Free Radical Scavengers." *J. Molecular Neuroscience*, 3:47–57.

Stadtman; Starke; Oliver; Carney; Floyd. "Protein Modification in Aging." Extracts 1992; 62:64–67 at the National Institutes of Health, Bethesda, MD.

Perricone, N. V. "Can Telomerase Provide a Cellular 'Fountain of Youth'?" *Skin and Aging* 6, no. 3: 16–18.

———. "What We Know about Telomerase and Skin Rejuvenation." *Skin and Aging* 7, no. 3: 15–18.

About the Author

Nicholas Perricone, M.D., received his degree in medicine from Michigan State University. His internship in pediatrics was completed at the Yale University School of Medicine and was followed by a residency in dermatology at the Henry Ford Medical Center in Detroit. Dr. Perricone is certified by the American Board of Dermatology and is a fellow of the New York Academy of Sciences. A clinical and research dermatologist in private practice in Connecticut, Dr. Perricone is an assistant clinical professor of dermatology at the Yale University School of Medicine. He is the author of numerous scientific articles and is a contributing editor to the peer-reviewed medical journal *Skin and Aging.* He is chairman of the International Symposium on Aging Skin, an annual meeting at which researchers come together from around the world to share their latest scientific breakthroughs in the prevention of aging and aging skin.

Dr. Perricone has been awarded 12 U.S. patents and dozens of related foreign patents based on his research and breakthrough technology in topical antioxidants and their ability to rejuvenate skin damaged by aging, the environment, health problems, or hormonal changes. NVPerricone Cosmeceuticals is the only skin care line researched, created, patented, and marketed by a board-certified dermatologist research scientist. *The Wrinkle Cure* is his first book.

For more information on N. Perricone, M.D., please visit his Web site at www.nvperriconemd.com.

The employees of Thorndike Press hope you have enjoyed this Large Print book. All our Large Print titles are designed for easy reading, and all our books are made to last. Other Thorndike Press Large Print books are available at your library, through selected bookstores, or directly from the publishers.

For more information about titles, please call:

(800) 223-1244
(800) 223-6121

To share your comments, please write:

Publisher
Thorndike Press
295 Kennedy Memorial Drive
Waterville, ME 04901